Compassionate Cities

Public health and end-of-life care

Imagine if communities really cared about their members' health and social well-being. Imagine if that care extended to the dying, death and loss experienced by everyone in those communities. Imagine if the idea of 'death' went beyond physical death and included the deaths of identity and belonging as experienced by those living with dementia or the aftermath of sexual abuse and dispossessed indigenous or refugee peoples. Such frameworks do partly exist in the World Health Organization's 'Healthy Cities' programs, but end-of-life care issues are often neglected. This book addresses these concerns and explores how compassion embraces empathy and support as new forms of 'health promotion'.

Beginning with an examination of the parallel histories of public health and end-of-life care, the book then critiques the limits of both. The theory and policy ideas of Healthy Cities are introduced and compared with those of Compassionate Cities, and the strengths and weaknesses of such large-scale programs are examined. The final sections of the book outline basic models of community development and strategies for implementing a Compassionate Cities program.

This is a book for practitioners who want to include end-of-life care issues or community development and health promotion ideas in their practices, and for anyone interested in social sciences, public health and end-of-life care. It argues that the integration of death, loss and compassion into contemporary public health ideas may address its limits and criticisms and help to create practical policies for future domestic and international well-being.

Allan Kellehear is a sociologist and Professor of Palliative Care at La Trobe University in Melbourne, Australia. In 2003–04 he was Visiting Professor of Australian Studies at the University of Tokyo, Japan. His previous works studying dying and its care include: *Dying of Cancer: The final year of life* (1990); *Experiences Near Death: Beyond medicine and religion* (1996); and *Health Promoting Palliative Care* (1999).

Compassionate Cities

Public health and end-of-life care

Allan Kellehear

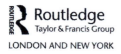

Routledge
Taylor & Francis Group

LONDON AND NEW YORK

First published in 2005 by Routledge
2 Park Square, Milton Park, Oxfordshire, OX14 4RN
Simultaneously published in the USA and Canada
by Routledge
29 West 35th Street, New York, NY 10001

Routledge is an imprint of the Taylor & Francis Group

© 2005 Allan Kellehear

Typeset in Sabon MT by J&L Composition, Filey, North Yorkshire
Printed and bound in Great Britain by TJ International Ltd,
Padstow, Cornwall

British Library Cataloguing in Publication Data
A catalogue record for this book is available from the British
Library

Library of Congress Cataloging in Publication Data
A catalogue record has been requested

ISBN 0-415-36772-7 (hbk)
ISBN 0-415-36773-5 (pbk)

In memory of the life and work of Miki Sawada
Magnum bonum

Acknowledgements

I would first like to thank my friend and colleague Ruth Beresford for patient and dedicated attention to the typing and formatting of this manuscript. A number of friends and colleagues have also provided critical feedback, suggestions for reading, and discussion opportunities to assist me in improving the arguments and evidence underlying this book.

I have benefited from Jan Fook's experience and interest in critical reflection, critical social work and postmodern writing. Michael Ashby has brought the considerable weight of his clinical experience in palliative medicine and his commitment to a wider social understanding of living and dying to ground my thinking in public health and palliative care. Likewise Patrice O'Connor gave me valuable feedback and encouragement on an earlier draft. Bruce Rumbold assisted me, as he always does, with readings in history and contemporary debates about palliative and pastoral care. Trevor Hogan and Paul Sinclair guided my reading in social theory and social role valorization, respectively. Ken Dempsey supported and guided my reading in community studies. I am also grateful for the support and enthusiasm for the idea of compassionate public health that I have received from Stuart Twemlow, my friend and colleague from the field of psychoanalysis.

All of these friends have helped me tread the fine line in emphasis that this kind of interdisciplinary book must negotiate between public health and palliative care, between vision, theory and practice issues, and between the importance of appreciative and critical observations. Although I have been committed to carefully negotiating these tensions, my attempts would have been much the poorer without the generous guidance of their criticism and feedback.

I extend my deepest thanks to each of them.

Contents

Preface

Death and loss continue to be misunderstood despite being the most universal and routine human experiences of all. For too long we have viewed death as the enemy of health when in fact it was illness and disease that properly occupied that place. We often identify death as a threat to or a failure of public health policies and initiatives. But this too is untrue.

The aim of all health care has always been to prevent *premature* death and *unnecessary* harm and to promote healing and well-being. In so far as death creates additional harm beyond itself, that impact is a necessary target for all good public health scholarship and practice. End-of-life care, in all its endlessly diverse expressions in daily life, is and should be the serious subject of public health investigation, policy and practice. The purpose of this book is to alert and help reorient public health to this universal set of human experiences.

The inevitability of death and the universality of loss are facts and meanings to understand. Their presence does not pass judgement upon our flimsy defences against them. Death and loss are experiences that challenge us to understand their role in shaping an individual's values and priorities, and through those personal alterations the very course of a nation's diversity of health experiences and histories. And all this goes on in every community, every day, this very moment, even as you read the words on this page.

From the personal experiences of dying, loss and grief to their subtle but strong presence in communities, or the living histories surreptitiously generated by them, or through further deaths that can be traced to earlier ones, the broader experience of death properly belongs inside – not outside – the gaze of public health. We have been slow to develop these public health insights. Sometimes we have even failed to recognize them at all.

Frequently we leave death and loss to the psychological professions and in this way support the falsity that death is an individual and private matter. Or we hand the problem of mortality to hospice and palliative care, giving them, and anyone else who looks on, the equally false impression that end-of-life care is merely terminal care, care in the final weeks and days of life. In these two professional storylines we no longer speak about the universality of loss or the commonplace ordinariness of death, dying and loss. And except for significant disasters, we seldom recognize every individual's death and loss as a community experience.

Consider the two following examples of how professional responses to end-of-life care currently shape and colour our everyday experiences and ideas about death and loss. In hospice and palliative care we frequently speak about 'whole person care' – the care devoted to the physical, psychological, social and spiritual dimensions of an individual life. But within the narrow confines of a health service so much of the attention to these aspects of a person is translated into occupational responses. We have doctors, nurses, social workers and counsellors. But sometimes these professions are viewed as inadequate to the complex needs of a person or their family, so yet more professions are recruited – massage therapists, aromatherapists, music therapists, pet therapists, occupational therapists or physiotherapists. And it doesn't end here either.

Every year more 'needs' of the dying person or their families are identified, analysed, debated or discussed in the academic and professional palliative care literature. This is followed by suggestions for yet other professionals to meet those needs – chaplains, pastoral care workers, family therapists, health-promotion workers or welfare workers. Where will the list end? Will it be a case of identifying the need then naming the professional? Can we afford to keep assembling – *should* we keep assembling – an occupational response to one person's life every time they do something as simple as enter a health service such as a hospice or palliative care programme?

If we do not find a way to recreate community involvement at the end of life this queue of professionals at the door of our homes and servicing our identities will see no end. Without a community involvement, professional involvement must become a rationalization and poor substitute for the multidimensional relationships that any one person enjoyed before encountering the local health service. The social and economic costs in permitting this 'professionalization' of death to continue are unimaginable.

But if palliative care has an explicit multidisciplinary response to death the field of grief and loss is somewhat less occupationally expansive, and yet this field has a more popular impact on public attitudes than palliative care. Recently two students were shot dead at one of the local universities in my city. I watched the television news coverage of the aftermath and was struck by a reporter's final observations in her report: 'Students and staff at the university are being provided with counselling'. I would like to live in a society where the first words about comfort and healing are recorded in the following way: '. . . and staff and students are now talking and commiserating with their friends and family'. But that will only ever happen, or happen with any surety, when we are confident that those friends and family know what to say and what to do in these circumstances, i.e. the circumstances of death and loss, expected or otherwise.

This book is about how we can begin to take those first steps towards regaining what was formerly unremarkably common – the community care of the dying and those living with loss. Although there are critical observations to be made in this book, it is not my intention to devalue the important work of counsellors or the necessary and pioneering work of palliative care in its work for people in the last weeks and days of life. Instead, I want to remind readers that community care around matters of death, dying and loss *preceded* professional care. I also want readers to remember that although modern professional care in these areas improves every day, that care remains unsupported, fragmented and incomplete without community involvement before, during and after these experiences.

The question of seamless social support for end-of-life care finds its answer, however ambitious and daunting the task, in community care. Questions of prevention, harm-minimization and aftercare issues find their fullest answer in community care. Yet where are the public health arguments and practice models for this type of community care and engagement?

Most of this book is devoted to a sketch for a theory of practice drawing upon the literature of community development, Healthy Cities and health-promoting palliative care. I outline what I term 'Compassionate Cities': a model of public health that encourages community participation in all types of end-of-life care.

Far from adding death and loss to the 'new' public health as a set of policy ideas, I argue that policies and practices inclusive of end-of-life care issues can be the basis of a radical reordering of priorities. A reordering of public health priorities that makes death and loss central to practice can build genuine empathy and this fact alone can re-energize any international and domestic programme of health reform.

I attempt to develop these arguments around the following nine chapters. I begin by tracing the social roots of organized care of the dying, comparing and contrasting professional care with community care from around the Middle Ages. I then compare the history of palliative care with the longer history of public health and medical care, and outline the conceptual and practice challenges for palliative care if it is to match those current developments in public health and to apply that care to their own work.

Later I examine three of the key pretenders to social and public health practices in end-of-life care – psychosocial palliative care, health-promoting palliative care and normalization theory. I describe why I believe these approaches are limited in their ability to develop a community focused public health approach to end-of-life care.

The middle parts of the book are devoted to outlining the theory, philosophy and policies of Compassionate Cities, linking these with their origins within the World Health Organization's Healthy Cities models and also addressing the critique of their shortcomings. Later chapters examine the social and political basis for embracing Compassionate Cities beyond their obvious fit with Healthy Cities approaches. I also provide a critical overview of the key problems I believe Compassionate Cities will face in the implementation and continuation of its programmes.

The final chapters provide some practice suggestions for implementation and action. Models for community development and professional involvement are rehearsed, as well as a range of suggestions that might initially be canvassed for community consideration. Unlike most of the earlier chapters these chapters are practical descriptions and suggestions for action.

The last chapter reflects on the broad debate about the future of public health. I describe where the ideas of compassion, the universality of loss and the idea of a broader understanding of death might fit into current public health priorities, and where their inclusion might address current anxieties and challenges for a global twenty-first century public health.

Chapter 1

The social roots of organized care for the dying

Modern thinking about end-of-life care is characterized by contradiction. When we imagine the end of life our thoughts quickly turn to the final days of dying. The ageing process, loss, violence, dispossession or simply living with a life-threatening illness rarely occupies much space in this understanding. Yet, ageing does involve significant confrontations with death and loss. Violence and dispossession cause experiences of loss and the deaths of people just as surely as do cancer or heart disease.

Whatever images we hold about dying, death or loss, our community images of these experiences also display yet other paradoxes. Community care of those dying or experiencing loss commonly evoke professional care images. We imagine medical care or other health services in general. We think in terms of pain control or counselling. Even here, the professional activities occur in hospitals, hospices or other treatment centres and professional locations. Our ideas about community care become so estranged, even confused, that we often accept *community based* care as a substitute, a mirage or as a theatrical lookalike for the real thing.

We struggle to imagine the police officer, the municipal councillor, the local school teacher or our own children as active and formal carers of people at the end of life. Instead, our images are of specialist health services and their personnel in hospice, palliative or nursing home care. In these simple ways, the social dimension of care – the way whole communities respond to end-of-life experiences and issues – becomes overly identified with medicine and their health service allies.

The history of health care has demonstrated that when we become totally reliant on professional services for our care several retrograde experiences come along for the ride. Firstly, we tend not to recognize, less use, the valuable resources and abilities that occur naturally among ourselves in all communities. Secondly, we tend to encourage others to define our needs in terms of their abilities to meet them. Finally, we tend to fail to develop partnerships that maximize the strengths of professional services with the strengths of community agency and action. How has this happened? How adequate are current professional responses, such as they are? Is there another way?

At the outset of this chapter, it is important to remind ourselves that we have always cared for our dying. In fact, the community care of the dying actually predates the history of professional care of the dying. Much of the strength and durability of that everyday care came from the general and targeted social supports and activities of whole communities towards their dying persons.

Too often we do not name the activity that is most important to living and dying. It is not medicines and holy oils that make us want to live, or die, in peace, but the social relationships and meanings of a personal lifetime. It is important to recognize that the history of travellers in the valley of the shadow of death is also a history of our *community care and support for each other*. Formal care of the dying has emerged gradually through history from that broader and longer history of community care.

Some of the professional care that emerged later did so from medical traditions – from physicians, surgeons or apothecaries. Some of the formal care came from other professional areas, from the spiritual traditions of care delivered by religious organizations. In these specific ways, organized 'professional' care of the dying has a long history in Western countries, particularly from medicine and religion. When pilgrimages became popular in fourth century Europe, for example, monasteries, convents, inns and hospices grew in number and importance along the roads leading to the Holy Lands (Kendall 1970).

Hospices specialized in care of pilgrims who were injured, fell ill or were dying. In fact, the modern hospital developed from their practices and organization (Bradshaw 1996). The Hospice at Jerusalem in about 1165, for example, contained about 2000 beds and experienced a daily death rate of about 50 patients (Sumption 1975: 199). Our popular understanding about care of the dying tends to be coloured by our repeated exposure to these above-mentioned kinds of observations. But organized care of the dying has been more than care by specialist practitioners from medicine and religion.

The social roots of our organized care of the dying have another, earlier and equally important, if less studied, source of care. This is the care we have given each other as ordinary citizens – as non-professionals if you like – and this care is a commonly overlooked chapter in our history of care towards the dying. Because modern ideas about community self-help within public health may trace its beginnings to these origins I will begin my review of the social roots of care of the dying from this rather neglected domain.

Community care

It has been a common observation by historians and sociologists that early physicians often confined themselves to cities and large towns where they were sought by the wealthier classes who could afford their solicitations (for European observations see Jewson 1976, for US observations see Starr 1982: 40). Medieval pilgrims, for example, died under the care of roadside hospices only because they were on pilgrimages that took them a long way from their doctors and further than their physical abilities or food rations would allow. But despite massive numbers of people who underwent these pilgrimages, particularly in so-called jubilee years declared by a pope (for example AD 1350) most people in the Middle Ages did not make pilgrimages. In fact, before the middle of the eleventh century these movements were composed of largely aristocratic individuals or small groups (Thompson 1928: 386), including many who were not typical peasant folk but 'beggars, thieves and prostitutes' (Herlihy 1997: 66).

More importantly, most people did not live in cities or large towns either. Rather, the majority of people in the Middle Ages lived in a settlement rather than migratory situation, and they lived that way mostly in rural settings, i.e. in small villages, hamlets or on family farms. Furthermore, when the majority of pilgrims returned from their journeys they returned to live and die in settlement circumstances. When common images of health care are adjusted for social class and regional specificity, the most common form of health care 'provider' in rural areas was probably a 'non-professional' (Gottfried 1983: 109). This was a person without formal training whose desire to help the sick gave them much experience and a few ideas swapped with other like-minded practitioners. In Europe some 15–20% of these non-professionals were women healers, and their fees were always the lowest and most affordable for the poor rural populations that they served.

Even in the USA, as late as the seventeenth and eighteenth centuries, all types of people took to providing health care to each other. Many of these people practiced health care while selling or conducting other businesses. Both men and women seemed to engage in these activities, particularly in poor, rural areas. As Starr (1982: 49) observed, 'In colonial America . . . most medical care was routinely provided by women in the home'. In the same work, Starr also noted that native Indian doctors were also popular. The interest in Native American Indian medicine was widespread and much respected by the early colonists of the USA.

There were also other periodic influences that led to a continuing marginal role for professional care of the dying. In European plague times, during the fourteenth and fifteenth centuries, a time when some 20–50% of the population were dying (Ziegler 1969, Platt 1996), few dying people were cared for by doctors or clerics, largely because so many of these professional carers were dead or dying themselves. Furthermore, many of the remaining clerics and physicians who were untouched by the plague were so terrified of the 'pestilence' that they refused to offer last rites or medical care to any of those affected by it. People were left to fend for themselves in any way they could, and in the company of anyone who was willing and brave enough to help them (Gottfried 1983: 78). Giovanni Boccaccio's account of the plague describes this problem in his much-quoted work *The Decameron*:

> Because of such happenings and many others of a like sort, various fears and superstitions arose among the survivors, almost all which tended toward one end – to flee from the sick and whatever had belonged to them. In this way each man thought to be safeguarding his own health . . . Meanwhile, in the midst of the affliction and misery that had befallen the city, even the reverend authority of divine and human law had almost crumbled and fallen into decay, for its ministers and executors, like other men, had either died or sickened, or had been left so entirely without assistants that they were unable to attend to their duties. As a result, everyone had to do as he saw fit.
>
> (Quoted from Gottfried 1983: 78)

Finally, we do well to remember that even in experiences of death that do not directly involve highly infectious diseases both clerics and doctors were merely one or two players included in a much larger cast of carers and participants. Aries (1974) and McManners (1985) both made the observation that dying was very much a public ceremony. Parents, friends, neighbours, servants and children, all of these parties were additional to the presence and involvement of men from medicine and the church. The dying were helped by these large groups, sometimes crowds from the local community, to meet their social obligations of making peace with family and community as well as God. The dying had a reciprocal set of obligations that locked him or her into a public morality play performed in several acts.

The cleric and the doctor often performed quite specific tasks for the dying person, but two sociological points are worth noting which help differentiate their former role with similar ones performed today. First, the conscious dying person was always the person in control. The dying person alone was chief organizer and arbiter of his or her final care and wishes. Professional services from church or medicine did not take charge in these kinds of settings. Although all the major elements of dying rituals were religious in origin and design, the home was not a formal institutional part of church. Secondly, although doctors and clerics played important roles these roles were played out alongside other equally important roles executed by others during the period of dying. Friends, servants, members of the wider community and family acted as prompts and supporters for death rituals. Often they played important roles as witnesses to confession, faith, social testimonials and personal legacies (McManners 1985: 234–69).

The higher the social standing of the dying person the greater the crowds, and the social diversity of those crowds, in helping the dying person perform these tasks. Servants required testimonials, lawyers required statements of legacy, Christians required affirmations of faith and confession. But in these ways and accounts, many of our best histories of death are also histories of bourgeois death. Because middle-class people were able to write, or were more often surrounded by those with writing ability, we know much about the community care and participation issues surrounding these social types of dying people.

Notwithstanding the debates about the empirical trustworthiness of various histories of death (Whaley 1981), the consistently middle-class and aristocratic images of dying in the Middle Ages suggests an additional dimension to the often exaggerated importance accorded to clerics and doctors. Professional players may have been minor, even absent, in many deaths among poor, rural residents. The middle-class emphasis in histories of dying is well illustrated by McManners (1985: 523) when he unobtrusively refers us to a mere footnote in the back of his epic *Death and The Enlightenment* to follow up details about what death was like for peasants – ironically the *majority* of the population.

But can this 'folk' or community care of the dying be regarded as an organized care? They most certainly can be regarded this way, especially if families are said to be economic and social organizations. As families are organized units of work and procreation they have always been the traditional guardians and midwives of birth and death among themselves. Furthermore, until quite recently health care has been seen as an additional family function rather than something regularly performed by and through public institutions and organizations. This is one key cultural and historical reason for the prominence of women in the caring professions today.

Finally, major life events, such as births, deaths and marriages, create organized responses for their social control and regulation. Cultures channel these functions through the rituals and customs exercised with public officials but in circumstances of community and household. Families perform these rituals and customs with or without public officials presiding over them. Such community response is always organized around traditional prescriptions. What forms does this style of care take today? What has happened to this community end-of-life care?

There are two major observations to make about the contemporary fate of community care. Firstly, the rise of the caring professions in the last 150 years or so (e.g. medicine, nursing, social work, or psychology) has meant the mass abdication and referral of community care concerns to these occupations. It is assumed that professionals mediate and express the care response for and by communities. This has led to a privatized and domestic understanding of community care. Community care becomes informal, privately motivated, a 'native' response to others in need. This might be a support role for the 'more appropriate' professional response to social and physical troubles of individuals and communities.

The widespread informal desire to be involved in care for others is channelled into formal organizations of care under the guidance or direct control of professionals. Volunteers, support groups and service clubs activities are all examples of how the informal desire to help translates into fund raising or other support duties bound for services or the direct management of professionals in them.

Secondly, contemporary end-of-life care has also become fragmented. Grief services and disaster planning operate largely independent of hospice services. Mainstream medical responses are frequently separated from the criminal justice system response to death and loss. Finally, the responsibility for all aspects of the dying experience has been, for example, delegated to hospice and palliative care services. Palliative care is defined as the social, spiritual, physical and psychological care of the dying person and their family. But how successful has the social dimension of this care been, and what form does it take today?

Hospice and palliative care

Whether for peasants or the wealthy, hospices during the Middle Ages continued to be places for pilgrims, travellers and the itinerant poor as an institutional form of care for the dying by religious organizations. In these places, clerics reigned supreme and they alone provided care for the dying in these settings. Their services continued more or less throughout the Middle Ages, paralleling the fluctuations of the fad for pilgrimage itself. And some of them even survived into the twentieth century performing similar functions for this particular group of people.

In Britain, for example, Anglican and Catholic religious organizations ran several hospices. However it must be emphasized that up to 1960 the British National Health Service had shown no commitment to terminal care provision in these or any other type of institutional setting (Clark 1999).

In 1967, Cicely Saunders established St Christopher's Hospice. Saunders was a nurse, medical practitioner and practicing Anglican, and is considered to be the founder of the modern hospice movement. Her interest in care of the dying was directed at people dying of cancer, an early informal emphasis that had wider implications for later policies. Gradually, the British government began to take over funding of hospice and palliative care services in Britain.

Overall then, it should be remembered that the modern palliative care movement grew from the thin traces of the only *specialist* tradition of care of the dying that made it into the twentieth century – the religiously inspired and managed hospices. Palliative care accepted death; viewing its professional challenge in terms of care within death's shadow.

On the other hand, post-plague medicine increasingly put its professional care energies into a somewhat opposite challenge – the fight against death itself (Illich 1976). In this way, modern medicine concentrated its professional efforts on models of care and types of interventions that might cure or prevent death. After all clinical efforts toward care failed, a doctor according to their personal abilities, would offer what psychological and social comfort they could. This professional space, or period of time, became the subsequent fertile ground for the resurgence of the modern hospice and palliative care movement.

Only in religious philosophies, rather than medical ones, was the problem of death part of the wider problem of a person's spiritual and physical journey through life. In the tradition of pilgrimage ideas, care of the soul was synonymous with whole person care, care of all aspects of a person's inner, social and physical life. Organized care of the dying as expressed in early hospice philosophy came to reflect these core pastoral values of care. These philosophies were ideological birthmarks pointing to their Medieval Christian origins.

Medieval beginnings of European hospice and palliative care began their modern consolidation in Britain in the 1960s, spread to North America in the 1970s and were supported by governments in Australia in the early 1980s (Rumbold 1998). Most of these hospice services were independent social experiments funded by private donations and staffed by idealist professionals and volunteers (Abel 1986). But such isolationism did not last long. Governments soon took over the planning and funding of palliative care services.

The desire by governments and health workers for end-of-life care that was patient-centred in terms of good symptom control, privacy and autonomy was expressed in numerous government reports, anecdotal and research-based articles in professional journals in the preceding decade of these developments (Clark 1999: 229–31). In the USA, the very survival of hospices depended on more reliable income sources to cater for professional employment and accommodation needs. Governments took a growing interest in hospice services just at a time when those services themselves questioned their own viability.

The gradual 'mainstreaming' of hospice and palliative care since the 1970s has generated a number of social observations of this form of care for the dying, many that appear to be critical of recent developments. It appears that the original holistic philosophy of hospice care of the dying is experiencing serious challenges and threats. Bradshaw (1996: 415) laments what she calls the 'secularization of the spiritual dimension', a process where the spiritual traditions derived from the Christian ethos are gradually diluted by a vague psychosocial mixture of New Age humanism and humanistic counselling. Pastoral traditions and ideas are being supplanted by the psychological and social sciences seeking to colonize new occupational terrain.

As early as 1983 Buckingham articulated the widespread hospice and palliative care ideal that whole person care meant that no one person can fully cater for the needs of the dying person and their family. This was an interdisciplinary project involving social workers, doctors, lawyers, nurses, clergy and many others from allied health professions. Yet the diversity of philosophies in publicly and privately run care programmes and the diverse levels of funding in these programmes mean that many services are highly idiosyncratic in their occupational priorities. Doctors and nurses seem to dominate, with social workers and pastoral care workers optional employees. In rural and remote areas, other occupations outside nursing may simply be used as referrals.

Rumbold (1998) warns of the immediate diluting effects of 'mainstreaming' palliative care services when these services must move away from emphasizing their distinctiveness and are pressured to rethink their common ground with other services. The concern about 'medicalization' has often been a vehicle for rehearsing concerns not simply about the professional emphasis of care – a legitimate concern in its own right – but also assumptions and attitudes to service delivery. Preferences for institutional settings and clinical interventions over community control and education are tied to these anxieties about medical power and ideology in palliative care.

Managed care, another style of health services mainstreaming, although with distinct benefits in cost control and interprofessional referral, tend to bring about these benefits by a provider-defined rather than purchaser-defined set of needs and priorities. The issue of cost–benefit can mute critical voices in palliative care (Abel 1986) by creating stronger links to hospitals and health services rather than communities, and by defining the problem of dying as 'end-stage care' rather than care of people living with life-threatening illnesses for whom cure is unlikely. In Australia, this can be observed in admission criteria for services defined by government funding bodies. Instead of palliative care being post-diagnostic care, palliative care is defined as care for people with a certain life expectancy, usually just weeks.

Several important implications follow from this recent government interest in care of the dying. Firstly, care of the dying is separated from care of the elderly. Palliative care was quickly identified as care of those dying from cancer. The funding criteria and cost-saving philosophies of government mean that palliative care is terminal care delivered by clinicians rather than quality-of-life care for people with life-limiting illnesses irrespective of life expectancy. Community involvement, such as it is, occurs through voluntary or fund-raising programmes. Volunteers underline and support the professional clinical care rather than serving as equal partners in that direct care.

Secondly, hospice and palliative care became a health services problem. This encouraged a shift of ideas about the responsibility for care from community to professional institutions. Services must think in terms of which professionals will be engaged, for what problem, for how long and at what cost when examining the problem of dying, death or loss in the communities in which they serve. Professionals are trained in clinical and bedside skills rather than ones in community development or public health.

Thirdly, to ensure funding criteria that are well defined, a fixed and determinate period of care is needed. Consequently, end-of-life care was defined in terms of life expectancy, usually the last weeks or months of life. End-of-life care became synonymous with palliative care, an unwarranted equation given that palliative care frequently confines itself to cancer care rather than broader problems of end-of-life care such as ageing or dementia care.

Fourthly, early hospice and palliative care leaders placed their faith, and their arguments about social change, on improved relationships between individuals, not on broad structural changes (Abel 1986: 81). Consequently, research and policy work within hospice and palliative care services rarely include public education, community development, and workplace, school and municipal partnerships. Dying, death and loss are defined as personal problems rather than targets of social change in community attitudes, values and behaviour. This reinforces the view that clinical rather than community skills should take priority in palliative care education and training.

Finally, although hospice care was originally defined by medieval and modern sources as whole person care – as care which embraced the physical, psychological, social and spiritual needs of the dying – these terms are now interpreted in clinical services terms. They merely refer to different *occupational groups* within the health service system and not to partnerships and activities in other public domains such as workplaces or schools. Palliative care is now 'team' care, *clinical* team care, i.e. the provision of doctors, nurses, social workers, or pastoral care or chaplancy.

The rapid and recent merging of a health service system response with a religious philosophy of care of the dying, although welcome and pioneering in many ways, must also be seen against the background of the greater progress of the wider health system approach to health and illness. There are ironies in this recent mainstreaming of palliative care with national health services. Clearly, palliative care services, research and policies have formed closer ties with clinical and institutional paradigms of care, and in so doing have inherited the medical emphasis on the importance of direct clinical interventions, particularly psychological and physical remedies.

The take up of links to public health medicine and community health nursing has been slow. In this way, palliative care is historically and professionally lagging behind in public health models of care. An even greater irony is that public health models are themselves reformist and holistic, making their policies and action strategies have great philosophical and political affinities with those of palliative care. Yet, professional discussions in palliative care journals and reports repeatedly show a consistent and conservative attraction to conventional biomedical and hospital-based resources, professions, partnerships and research priorities. Although these are very much the mainstream values of medicine itself, both the history of medicine and current medical directions demonstrate a greater role, respect and involvement with explicitly social models of care through a commitment to public health. I will describe and examine that involvement below.

Public health and medical care

Numerous social and historical observers have noted how the Western medical system, for example, has responded to the changing disease burden brought by modernity (see Waddington 1973, Jewson 1976, Torrens 1978, Starr 1982, Najman 2000). The last 150 years of Western history has seen several dramatic shifts in our epidemiology and health care responses.

Most of human history has been characterized by short life expectancies, high rates of infectious disease morbidity and mortality, and absent, poor or inadequate professional care. However, for 99% of that history our social and economic systems were of the hunter-gatherer type, where the burden of infectious diseases was probably lower than when we developed into agrarian settlement societies (Powles 1973). Settlement societies, at least until the late eighteenth century, encouraged a higher birth rate, a narrower range of nutritional choices, and a greater build up of human and animal waste and parasites. In these close quarters, any infections spread far more easily. But despite persistent myths to the contrary, it was not direct medical care that improved the health of modern people. Rather, it was social and economic gains that altered the lifestyles and hence health of industrial peoples.

Powles (1973) argues that recent developments in birth control, immunization, surgery, pain and other symptom controls have improved the quality of life of modern people, and have contributed to the control of recent mortality rates. These contributions however are much overrated when compared to the role of public health. The bulk of the lowered mortality enjoyed in the nineteenth and twentieth centuries has come more directly and dramatically from public health measures. Improved sanitation and nutrition, stemming from a gradual rise of economic prosperity in industrialized societies, are believed to be chiefly responsible for these improvements.

Indeed, McKeown (1971: 36) argues that clinical medical care was not significant in increasing the general population's health until the 1920s or 1930s. Even when examining the role of antibiotics, Powles, quoting from a 100-year review by Porter (1972), observed that 90% of the decline in mortality from scarlet fever, diphtheria, whooping cough and measles from 1860 to 1965 occurred *before* the introduction of antibiotics or immunization programmes.

During and after the Industrial Revolution and until the mid-twentieth century, we developed a mixed burden of disease that resulted from improved public living conditions and the development of widespread, research-based medical care. Life expectancies rose sharply. Technological innovations and interventions became dramatic, less life threatening and therefore more attractive to individuals and governments. The arrival of infection control, anaesthesia and X-rays in the late nineteenth century increased the use and value of surgery (Starr 1982: 156). After the Second World War, the discoveries of science, such as radar, the atom bomb and penicillin, dramatically raised the status, public profile and the funding level to science. As Starr (1982: 336) so eloquently puts it, 'At home the advance of science and medicine, like economic growth, offered the prospect of improved well-being without requiring any profound re-organization of society.'

But chronic diseases such as cancer and circulatory diseases began to overtake infectious diseases as leading causes of death, and antibiotics were useless against these new troubles. In the first flushes of success and idealism about science from the Second World War, governments and popular opinion became increasingly focused on the idea of cure – what many commentators have described as an obsession with 'magic bullets' (Dubos 1959). Enormous funding was dedicated to medical and pharmacological research and the development of hospitals in all the major industrial countries.

As it became highly apparent during the 1960s that the prospect of cures for illnesses such as cancer or heart disease were not going to be available in the short-term, medical care re-engaged with the question of social behaviour and choices. A prevention strategy was needed. The research and policy attention that local governments had given to 'first-wave' public health issues that lowered infection rates during the previous one hundred years began to be rethought in terms of the challenges posed by these new chronic conditions.

Early first-wave public health had great successes during its campaigns against 'dirt and filth' but its self-definitions consistently brought it into disrepute and conflict with conventional medical care. Public health as the striving for health by community efforts was always bound to bring it into conflict with other institutions such as medicine, and to raise questions about the role of state intervention and individual rights, particularly in the USA. What was true for medicine in these concerns was also true for issues of national social welfare in that country: 'It was a cardinal principle in America that the state should not compete with private business' (Starr 1982: 196). In the middle years of the twentieth century public health took a back seat to the worldwide desire for the 'technological fix' from science and medicine.

But in the 1970s the upward spiral in health care costs seemed endless, most of which covered the growth of hospitals, developments in new drugs and technologies, and the costs of medical education and personnel. Finally, these ever-increasing national economic burdens gave governments everywhere reason to pause. This was also coupled with increasing evidence of questionable health gains and cost-effectiveness against the key disorders that plagued modern people – cancer and heart disease. Rather ironically, the re-emergence of a new infectious disease during the 1980s, a disease which did not respond to antibiotics or antiviral agents, also turned medical and public health observers to re-examine the idea of prevention. With the rapid worldwide spread of AIDS (acquired immune deficiency syndrome), public health gained a new ascendancy and renewed support.

The so-called 'new public health' (or the second wave of public health initiatives) was a phrase applied to a public health approach reliant on personal and community education. This differentiated it from earlier first-wave approaches that concentrated on sanitation or isolation and disinfection (Starr 1982: 191). The new public health of the 1970s and 1980s expanded the idea of personal and community education by actively involving the state in public education and community development campaigns in all major areas of social life. Hazards such as tobacco use, shared needles, overeating, sedentary lifestyle or exposure to hazards such as asbestos or ultraviolet light to the design of automobiles and workplaces came into the public health gaze. All of these areas and more were targets of strategies for the avoidance of hazards that may be associated with them.

Many of these strategies began their life as *behavioural* strategies, i.e. emphasizing personal change, but it soon became obvious that this approach blamed the victim. Not everyone was capable of changing his or her environment or habits. *Social* approaches to public health were needed. Workplaces might need modification as well as work practices. Cars may need redesign as well as their drivers encouraged to think about alcohol use and driving. People need to be educated about the life-threatening implications of smoking but tobacco companies may need to carry warnings on their products. Many of these second-wave public health approaches came to be known as 'health-promotion' efforts.

From the early 1980s – about the time that palliative care services were attracting initial interest from the Australian government – the World Health Organization (WHO) had been leading a campaign to introduce health-promotion ideas into the health practices and policies of all willing nations. For example, nations such as Australia, the USA and Britain now take for granted that no fully adequate health response to cancer, AIDS or heart disease can be said to be taken by a country if that response is confined to health services and tertiary interventions. Health is everyone's responsibility. Healthy communities are ones where employers, governments, churches, schools and workplaces support safety and health through early interventions and prevention programmes and health service partnerships with the community.

Although much public health in wealthy countries such as the USA or UK remain medically dominated in their funding and practice priorities (see Beaglehole and Bonita 1997), there continues to be a basic recognition and commitment to community approaches and partnerships to health care beyond simple service provision.

End-of-life care: the challenge for all communities

Read against these broader changes in our understanding of health, the recent developments in palliative care services can be seen as welcome but currently limited to a pre-1980s health system response. Clearly, end-of-life care is more than care for terminal cancer patients. The need to address end-of-life care for others in other disease groups and those in aged care facilities pose a funding, policy and practice challenge for all of us in health care.

The prevailing view that a service response, i.e. a solely clinical palliative care response, is an adequate main response to end-of-life care is in need of major re-examination and revision. Planning a public health response to end-of-life care is clearly important in recapturing an earlier vision of hospice care as whole person, community care.

Finally, early intervention strategies need to be developed and theorized, not only as important adjuncts to ideas about physical symptom control but also more crucially in terms of social, psychological and spiritual care responses. The idea that many of these social, psychological or spiritual issues can be addressed in the final weeks or months is out of step with the personal realities. The catastrophic psychosocial impact of diagnosis or reoccurrence of disease (Dudgeon et al 1995) demands that any professional or community response to these troubles must begin here, at the earliest point of personal recognition of the health threat.

The need for public health policy and practice responses in palliative care is important for complementing existing clinical services. They are also important in expanding and diversifying those services so that the challenge of whole person care can be met by the creative fullness of our modern responses to health care. This must include partnerships with communities. But what would a social response to end-of-life care look like? What themes and lessons to guide us should we take from past social experiences of organized care of the dying?

From our perusal of the past care of the dying we can discern seven major themes that reoccur in these historical and cultural descriptions. Community care of the dying has repeatedly demonstrated, until quite recently, two important social lessons.

Firstly, care of the dying throughout our past has been a NORMAL AND ROUTINE matter for families and communities. In pre-industrial times this sense of the normal and routine came with significant experience of death and loss. Today, direct, personal experiences of death are rare, although direct personal encounters of loss are arguably not so rare. Nevertheless, where experience cannot guide or give confidence to communities, education potentially can. There is an important role for public education in the normalization and routinization of the modern experiences of death.

Secondly, past patterns of community care have illustrated the importance of COMMUNITY RELATIONSHIPS in that care. This has been de-emphasized today, perhaps because it is a critical distraction to our current dependence on professional services or perhaps because current social histories of dying seem preoccupied with bourgeois death. Whatever the reason, clearly palliative care professionals cannot embark upon these new challenges alone and unassisted. Policy development, workplace changes, school education and public education, just to name a few of the examples of a public health approach, will need expertise and experience from a wide range of people and institutions. Professionals will be important to any public health approach to end-of-life care but they will be, as they have been in the past, part of a much larger cast of actors.

The history of hospice and palliative care has repeatedly highlighted two further issues. Firstly, that care of the dying person must be WHOLE PERSON CARE. From medieval pastoral traditions that we can trace to European pilgrimages, palliative care views care of people at the end of life as not simply in terms of symptom control, e.g. of control over pain and breathlessness, but psychological, spiritual and *social* supports. A person is not merely a body (or a patient) but a citizen, a person intricately connected to a community of friends, family and co-workers, and also the values and belief systems of that community. The good death has always been a reflection of the good life, and these moral ascriptions have no meaning outside the social context of the dying person as citizen and the networks that underpin that social identity and experience.

This is the key reason why THE FAMILY IS A BASIC UNIT OF CARE in hospice and palliative care and not simply the 'individual'. This is the second theme that emerges from palliative care literature, both clinical and historical. Palliative care services have tended to approach care of the dying person and their family. This is long-standing recognition that individuals are part of a social system that cannot be arbitrarily divided during any professional intervention without serious consequences to the health, morale and well-being of that person. At the core of this simple revision of a health care target – from patient to family – is the reaffirmation of an old public health ideal. Good medical science is social science.

The history of medical care has shown that an equally important power of modern medicine is to be found in joint scientific and community efforts towards achieving health. That partnership is now known as 'public health' and three themes emerge from the public health efforts to improve health.

First, the INVOLVEMENT OF THE STATE has been shown to be crucially important. Clinical interventions are not adequate for the task of health maintenance and illness prevention, or for the need for mass screening and treatments for disease burdens at population level. Antibiotics can control small infectious outbreaks but national public health measures ensure that such outbreaks, when they do occur, have minimal national impact.

Secondly, THE IDEA OF PREVENTION – as an adjunct and alternative idea to cure – has been crucial to any effective programme of attack in all diseases, and social and physical hazards that may impact on the health and safety of individuals and large populations. There is much we can do for road trauma victims in an emergency department of a hospital but if we wish to minimize or eradicate this problem in the first place we need to think about prevention. Prevention is an early intervention strategy that may involve more than medical activities and policies. It may need the assistance of government, business and schools. Without prevention, medical care is not health care but simply care when things go wrong.

Finally, both partnerships with the state, and the development of ideas and actions towards the goals of prevention, necessarily mean that health care – any form of health care – must go BEYOND MERE SERVICES. Health care is about healthy environments and relationships and these, when they are effectively supported by our key institutions, promote healthy bodies and minds.

The above seven themes – normalization, community relationships, whole person care, the person as social unit, state involvement, prevention and the need to go beyond health services ideas – are the instrumental building blocks of any public health approach to end-of-life care. They also underlie all the most positive aspects of our care of dying people down through Western history, from its sources in the community and to those from the healing professionals in churches of God or science. They provide a balance to clinical and custodial approaches to care and are consistent with several observations about end-of-life care today.

Firstly, the longer part of dying occurs outside the home. If dying is about living, loving and working with a life-threatening illness until one can no longer do so, we recognize that the longer part of that lifestyle occurs outside formal health care institutions and outside 'care and treatment episodes'.

Secondly, although many people die in hospices and hospitals, an equal or greater number also die in nursing homes and retirement villages. Outside of the industrial countries of the world, even more people simply die in ordinary villages of every kind around the globe. In these contexts, particularly in industrial settings, we are yet to relearn the old ways of caring for one another – those persons who are dying and also those left behind. For others who know these ways, we are yet to document, examine, adapt and translate these experiences into social insights that can benefit us all, irrespective of the cultural settings from which they originate.

Thirdly, end-of-life care is more than palliative care. Every day people die in road traumas, suicides, and homicides, and disasters take people in hundreds and thousands at a time. Aside from death from old age, there are also tolls of death from the political and social plight of indigenous peoples all over the world. From civil wars to the negative health effects of dispossession, our current understandings about caring for those dying and experiencing loss have yet to be inclusive of these people and contexts.

Death is inevitable and loss is universal. These two great human experiences are obviously not addressed in their manifold expressions by current models of palliative care, and will not be if this specialist health field confines itself to clinical and acute care methodologies. A public health approach is the only approach with the epistemological, political and scientific tools to complement palliative care social philosophy, and also to take it forward and beyond its current clinical definitions and sites.

And public health, as an interdisciplinary scientific concern, cannot continue to ignore dying, death and loss – experiences that are not merely experiences to postpone. Death and loss are also experiences and events open to harm-minimization and they can be springboards to positive personal and social growth. Loss itself has a morbidity and mortality burden that can be counted and described not simply in physical and psychiatric terms but in social, moral and economic ones too. In science and art, in sickness and health, citizens and professionals must, sooner rather than later, confront the universal challenge that we *can* face death constructively, if the national, community and personal will is there.

In the next chapter I will examine the key social and health-promotion approaches to end-of-life that have been attempted and would-be pretenders to this mantle of public health care of the dying. So how adequate is the competition?

Chapter 2

Current approaches to end-of-life care

In this chapter I examine current social approaches to end-of-life care and ask: are they public health ones? Although palliative care does not currently embrace a formal public health practice in its approach to end-of-life care it does attempt to integrate a basic social understanding of care. The most common form of this understanding is in the interest that palliative care displays in 'psychosocial' care. It is here, in the professional interest in areas such as policy, service development, psychology, communication and family support, that palliative care champions the 'social'.

Furthermore, the social dimension of care is given special occupational support through the hiring of professionals such as social workers or counsellors. Recent broad policy statements by special institutes or peak bodies representing palliative care also frequently employ the language of community and society. But the hallmarks of a true public health policy and practice are at least defined in their basic commitment to education, community development and state involvement. In these ways, can the psychosocial approach in contemporary palliative care be regarded as a genuinely public health one?

I have recently outlined a theory of health-promotion practice for palliative care (Kellehear 1999a) that aimed to integrate basic public health ideas into the clinical service approach. Clinical services might transform some of their offerings into community offerings; empower patients and their families by taking an early intervention approach to social and spiritual issues around dying and loss; or add education functions to those of treatment, palliation and support. But does a health-promoting palliative care approach adequately address end-of-life care in its broadest community sense? Does a health-promoting palliative care adequately guide us to a programme of community care led by that community, or is this merely expanding our understanding of clinical work with the dying and their families? Does health-promoting palliative care merely turn this style of public health into yet another 'clinical service' performed ON the community rather than something BY the community?

There are other more radical suggestions for end-of-life care too. 'Normalization' theory, otherwise known as 'social role valorization' theory, describes ways that a society may organize itself so as to prevent marginalization of citizens, or roles that are considered 'spoilt' or are of lower social value to others. Much of the political energy around deinstitutionalization movements in psychiatry and disability have at their theoretical core this idea of normalization. How relevant are these ideas to end-of-life care? Can these ideas offer us a basis for theorizing community care practices at the end of life that embrace or even surpass current public health ideals?

I will begin this chapter by briefly outlining the main concepts and principles of public health – the who, why and how of public health practice. Employing these assumptions, I will review the occupational and policy limits to psychosocial palliative care. I will then describe health-promoting palliative care and raise critical questions about the design limitations of any set of health-promotion ideas that attempt to embed themselves in the context of a clinical approach. Finally, I will review normalization theory and assess the value and efficacy of this approach as an alternative to an outright public health one.

What is public health?

Any examination of the public health literature will reveal a diverse set of definitions of public health. Broadly speaking, public health policies and initiatives include *all* organized efforts to control and improve the health of national or regional populations (Tulchinsky and Varavikova 2000: xix). These wide-ranging possibilities can include the hospital system, direct medical services and other professional health services, but also less obvious programmes such as purification and fluoridation of the water supply, the development and enactment of laws regarding drug use (medical and recreational), burial and cremation, automobile and work safety, to other community programmes such as immunization, food handling safety and the control of pests that endanger human health such as fleas or rats.

However, the term 'public health' is more commonly used in a narrower sense to cover early and later initiatives and objectives to combat the major disease burdens of a society. In these uses of the term, there are frequently historical distinctions and debates about the 'old' first-wave public health and the so-called 'new' second-wave one. The first-wave public health initiatives, particularly in the West, were more concerned with sanitation efforts, the procurement of fresh water supplies and the containment of infectious diseases. The more recent second-wave public health approaches are often identified with health-promotion issues of public education, especially where this applies to lifestyle issues of diet, harmful substances in the environment such as tobacco or asbestos, and health and safety in the workplace.

Of course, such distinctions are not only arbitrary they also ignore the fact that the 'old' public health approaches are alive and well today. These approaches are relevant and active in the poorer nations of today, indigenous communities in the wealthier ones, as well as reinventing themselves in new infectious disease problems such as AIDS or hepatitis C (Beaglehole and Bonita 1997).

It is also the case that issues of sanitation and infection control are not mere mechanical issues related to the identification of sources of fresh water or supplying clinical interventions for disease outbreaks. ALL public health involves an educational component, a community effort and a government role in one capacity or another, either through legislative changes, support or surveillance activities of one kind or another. In these obvious ways, we can speak comfortably about a single understanding of public health. This definition has the following characteristics:

> Public health is a concern with social efforts led by government and actioned by communities, often in partnerships with health and other social organizations, to lessen disease and/or improve health at the broadest population level. These efforts occur through education, improvement of social capital and community development, enactment of laws, partnerships with health services and professionals, and the creation of safe and sustainable social and physical environments.

Historically, it is governments that have led public health initiatives. National governments or local council or municipal governments have developed policies, provided funding or personnel or education or information campaigns to spur communities into action over one or several health or disease issues within the orbit of their authority. Few campaigns can hope to succeed without community support, for the epidemiology of the problem is so wide or the populations affected so extensive that community action is vital to any strategy towards the solution. Various strategies have included education at schools, churches, workplaces or in homes, employing all media at a government's disposal – print, radio, television and Internet, employing advertising and/or explicit warnings or information. Sometimes laws have been important to the success of certain safety campaigns, e.g. drink-driving laws, or others concerning helmet use at work or riding bikes, or the display of health warnings on cigarette packaging.

Also important to public health approaches to health care is the improvement of 'social capital'. This idea assumes that a community that interacts with itself frequently is also one with high levels of trust, social support and community morale, which fosters interest in matters that affect their community, friends, family or workmates. A community with significant social capital is a community interested in its own health and welfare. When these levels are not strong, community development strategies may be important in building social capital.

Community development concerns practical efforts to bring community members together to build trust and interest in health and safety. Neighbourhood Watch, community gardens, child safety house schemes or festivals are all examples of community development which evoke a sense of belonging and interest in one's place of living. The need to build partnerships – to work for, design toward and support health and well-being – is crucial to successful, modern paths to public health. We work *with*, not *on*, communities.

The mobilization of community to act on its own needs is often prompted by public health information about the prevention of disease or knowledge about health maintenance. Communities can be spurred on to act when new information is received from medical or safety authorities. At the level of knowledge dissemination and professional support of community practices, partnerships between community and health services can be crucial to the development and sustainability of community initiatives.

The creation of safe and sustainable environments has been a long tradition in public health. Public health initiatives target physical and social settings. Examples range from simple matters such as access to safe and sustainable sources of drinking water to a social and legislative environment where workplace safety is upheld as a vital value and attitude in all occupations. But these environments may also extend to social environments that encourage better nutrition and lower stress levels for people. Optimal health messages may heighten awareness about dietary control and shopping preferences, and lowering stress could lend itself to community programmes to raise awareness of domestic abuse or workplace bullying. How do such processes and ideas make their presence felt in contemporary palliative care?

Psychosocial palliative care

As I argued in the last chapter, palliative care has recently evolved into a clinical set of disciplines whose emphasis and professional investment has been in the development of health services, interventions and professional relationships based on narrow ideas of expertise and patient identification.

End-of-life care is now increasingly synonymous with palliative care, i.e. the idea of caring for those who will die soon from a progressive, incurable disease, particularly but not exclusively cancer. Ageing and dying have little conceptual or practical overlap in services or the research literature in palliative care. And the palliative care interest in the development of health services has led to a concern over types of these services and the sites where these might be relevant. Whether in-patient or home-based, or medical or pastoral services, or whether these are useful or affordable to hospices, nursing homes or in situations of respite care, the emphasis is solidly on services and sites.

As one would expect from such a health services orientation, the research and practice emphasis has been in the development and execution of treatment intervention. The practical professional concern and task has been with symptom control. These symptoms can be physical or psychological. Furthermore, the social relationships in this form of end-of-life care are characterized by professionalization of relations. Professionals in palliative care 'know' about end-of-life care and people who enter the orbit of their care become 'patients' or 'clients'. However 'patient-centred' the approach to that care, the person at the centre of it becomes merely a site for services.

The idea of the life of a citizen – that a dying person may have needs more complex and beyond health services for the majority of his or her time whilst living with a life-limiting illness – is rarely considered a time or experience for palliative care to make a contribution. Only when things become 'problems' – physical, psychological, social or spiritual – does palliative care as a health service become active. In this way, the psychosocial aspects of palliative care are problem-seeking or problem-based. They also emphasize professional expertise and patient experiences, and ignore the person as citizen and community member. The sites of interest to palliative care are the custodial ones in health care; the hospices, hospitals, nursing homes or home care 'teams'. Community exists only in so far as this is a site for public education or patient residence.

As citizens, people are capable of self-help and, as in other stages of life aside from death, are able to call upon and use the resources of support, information and power inherent in their communities. These communities, in their turn, have relationships with various governments, and partnerships with health and social organizations that have a bearing on their everyday well-being and health, and logically, their experiences of dying and loss. The clinical services characteristics of contemporary palliative care are best illustrated by their current understanding of self-help groups; the occupational response to psychosocial care; and recent policy statements about challenges now facing palliative care.

One of the most intriguing interpretations of self-help is the common view that this is synonymous with the development or existence of support groups (Gray 2001). Several interesting observations should be made about this conflation or identification of self-help with support groups. Firstly, self-help is ironically interpreted as help for the *individual* self by joining illness- or disease-specific support groups. The idea of communities helping themselves deal with dying, death or loss, i.e. community self-help, is absent.

Secondly, these groups are literally psychosocial groups – groups that deal in talk and information, and the development of close interpersonal support for one another and their circle of intimates. The idea of self-help in death and dying expressing itself in political or lobby groups is not dealt with in the palliative care literature and yet such groups have existed in the HIV/AIDS area, for example. These lobby groups have also helped to speed access to new treatments, to lobby governments to change laws that have prevented access to patient records, or to include victim statements in court cases involving homicide. Other self-help groups have helped to raise the profile of the citizen's plight in matters to do with grief and bereavement (e.g. Mothers Against Drink Drivers). The broader community aspects of self-help are bypassed and the broader idea and social movement is interpreted narrowly in terms of a treatment intervention organized by non-professional groups.

Thirdly, despite the narrow view of self-help as support groups, as groups of people banding together to maximize information and support for each other, these groups quickly become understood as 'patient' support groups. 'Patients', rather than 'citizens' with rights and agency, or as people who do as they please according to their own vision of the world and within the prevailing law, have duties and obligations to health professionals. By defining people as patients, people can then be viewed as compliant or non-compliant, as needing guidance and help from professionals, or as people who overidentify with their physical or psychological problem. This characteristic leads to the fourth.

At least some of the academic and professional literature expresses a concern that these 'patient' support groups may be breeding grounds for misinformation, malcontents, criticism of the health care system or some of its members, and may contribute to inappropriate attitudes such as false hope and interest in alternative therapies (Gray 2001: 55). In other words, some patient groups can foster delinquency, non-compliance and outright criticism, as well as positive functions of support and education.

In these above ways, we can see psychosocial palliative care interpret a simple social arrangement of people coming together to help each other in the most narrow way possible. The self-help group becomes the support group, the support group becomes the patient group, and concerns about 'bad' patients or 'outcomes' soon arise and become identified with these developments and structures. But support groups are not the only type of psychosocial care that is of interest or is offered by palliative care.

There are occupations within palliative care that are concerned with psychosocial matters. Chief among those occupations is social work and counselling. It is both a comment on the clinical nature of palliative care and the perceived relative importance of psychosocial care in palliative care that, in Australia at least, not all palliative care services have these occupations on their payroll. Those palliative care services that do employ social workers or counsellors have these as recent employees, as fractional employees, or as non-specialist referrals from other services. This precarious state of affairs notwithstanding, what community activities are these workers engaged in?

Some recent articles in the *Journal of Palliative Care* and *Palliative Medicine* provide some of the first research-based clues on what these professions provide dying persons and their families. A content analysis of the themes that emerged from a study of the job activities of counsellors in Canada revealed that these occupations played no community role whatsoever (Thompson et al 2001). The list of activities included 'companioning', assessment, planning and evaluation, counselling interventions, facilitating and advocacy, patient and family education, consultation and reporting, and team support.

A similar study of social work in palliative care in the UK (Sheldon 2000) revealed that 'social' in social work in that country appeared to be work with clients, family and other professionals on 'the team'. Outside the specifics of family and household, social worker Sheldon (2000: 494) describes social workers influencing the environment as 'advice and information giving' or 'liaising' or 'supporting external colleagues'. No understanding of a social world beyond family and household is present to permit a professional imagination or practice of health promotion or broader public health ideas. Social workers and counsellors, like doctors and nurses in palliative care, are face-to-face clinical workers for whom community, citizenship or self-help are but distant or absent dimensions of health care. But what about the articulated statements about future challenges and possibilities in palliative care? Are there echoes of an interest or commitment to public health ideas in these new developments?

The USA has produced at least two recent and important national statements about end-of-life care policy. *Last Acts* is a national campaign initiated by the Robert Wood Johnson Foundation (Task Force on Palliative Care 1998, Cassel and Demel 2001). *Last Acts* articulates a set of 'precepts' that include ideas about: (1) respecting patient goals, preferences and choices; (2) comprehensive caring; (3) utilizing the strengths of interdisciplinary resources; (4) acknowledging and addressing caregiver concerns; and (5) building systems and mechanisms of support. These precepts have no concepts of community, citizenship or policy concepts that include those ideas. All precepts are articulate about services, and occupational and institutional responses to end-of-life care (which they identify as palliative care), and all precepts speak of people as patients. People are not multiroled human beings with agency.

Although the precepts argue for the need for 'systematic reform . . . within society' (p 109) these reforms refer to issues of access to services, professional education, financial reform around Medicare and professional development issues for palliative care itself. Rather depressingly, 'community' resources are described in terms of '. . . hospitals, home care, hospice, long term care, adult day services' (p 111).

The presence of any interest in public health policy development is nowhere present. The desire to mobilize community participation in end-of-life care is nowhere present. The *Last Acts* precepts are about service sector and professional development, not community development. The barriers to palliative care can be surmounted if palliative care were made into palliative medicine (Cassell and Demel 2001: 436); if changes in Medicare allowed greater patient access; if more education were provided for health professionals; and if the general public were encouraged to think of end-of-life care in terms of providers, and the problems and barriers that they encounter.

The Institute of Medicine (1997) in its policy monograph *Approaching Death* holds out greater hope for a public health sensitivity, but does remain chained to a narrow understanding of the social and the community. Its recommendations describe commitment to a vision where everyone should be entitled to quality palliative care. Health professionals must commit to improving care for 'patients' and there must be system reform. Everyone from policy-makers to consumer groups to 'purchasers' should encourage measurement of quality of life and sound programme outcomes.

Health care organizations should be held accountable for their service offerings and there should be drug prescription reform around the use of opioids. Palliative care should be included in more health professional education. Palliative care should become a medical specialty. There should be research development in the field of palliative care. Finally, but most importantly for the purposes of public health, there should be greater public discussion of improved understanding of dying and loss and community obligations about end-of-life care.

This final recommendation is the first policy document of recent times to mention community obligations around end-of-life care. It occurs alongside an equally encouraging section on 'Whole Community Model of End-of-Life Care' (Institute of Medicine 1997: 10). Unfortunately, a closer inspection of that model reveals a greater interest in service sector issues than the community itself. There is a major interest in the development of services and custodial environments such as hospices and home care.

There is further interest in the development of professional personnel and protocols that support service delivery and quality control with it. Finally, the 'whole community' model of care expresses an interest in support systems in the workplace, churches and other institutions, and public education to improve awareness, encourage 'advanced planning' and provide informational resources for emotional, spiritual and practical end-of-life care.

This policy document moves palliative care into a positive language and set of ideas about the community basis of end-of-life care that promises to recognize community power and resources in supporting the dying, death and loss experiences of its members. But once again, a close scrutiny of that language tends to reveal a conservative and narrow interpretation of the social. Social activities and ideas are not described in terms of community

actions beyond 'practical' support. That practical support is about mobiliz-
ing the community to facilitate or develop a support structure that will
allow people who are dying to maintain a satisfactory contact with health
services.

The language and ideas of citizenship, health care partnerships, and of
investments in social capital and community development are nowhere
articulated or explored. The active development of ideas that might create
visions of social or cultural environments that are supportive and sustainable,
government policies that facilitate those environments, and the suggestions
for public education and legislation to cement those innovations are
nowhere to be seen.

In these ways, psychosocial palliative care is not public health end-of-life
care because its definition of the community is marginal, its idea of person-
hood barely goes beyond the idea of the patient, and because its policy
development is hopelessly committed to self-interested notions of service
sector and professional development rather than community development
and citizen participation. A minor departure from these concepts and
parameters is the idea of health-promoting palliative care.

Health-promoting palliative care

In 1998, the Victorian State Government in Australia funded the La Trobe
University Palliative Care Unit in the School of Public Health (Kellehear
1999a, 1999b). This is a demonstration project designed to explore, adapt,
evaluate and disseminate health-promotion strategies for possible adoption
by clinical palliative care services (Kellehear 2003). In 2003 the national-
lead organization for Australian palliative care, Palliative Care Australia
recognized public health initiatives in palliative care as one of 11 'essential
elements' in their service system alongside respite care, continuity and coordination of care, and bereavement support (Palliative Care Australia 2003).
I have discussed the main philosophical and theoretical ideas behind the
Unit and its current work elsewhere (Kellehear 1999b; 2003; 2004) but
summarize these below.

The underlying philosophy of health-promoting palliative care is the
World Health Organization's (WHO) Ottawa Charter for Health
Promotion (WHO 1986, Kellehear 1999b). This charter outlines five major
philosophical principles behind the need to support and maintain health in
communities. These are: building public policies that support health; creating supportive environments; strengthening community action; developing
personal skills; and reorienting health services.

These principles underline the deeper view that health care should be
participatory, not something we *do to others* but a style of health care that
we *do with others*. The charter also recognizes the essentially *social*
character of health and illness. Most health and illness is not a random and

idiosyncratic phenomenon. It is well understood that *environmental condi-tions* shape and promote some types of biological responses over others. Poor living conditions, poor nutrition, lack of sewerage systems or unclean drinking water all promote infectious diseases. Poor contraceptive beliefs and practices create population pressures. Tobacco use or poor protection against ultraviolet light can promote some types of cancer. Health and illness are social experiences.

Because health promotion also recognizes the social character of health and illness, education, information and policy development in health care is crucial to the security, safety and health of all communities. Such pro-grammes are designed for the well and the ill, so that we maximize the conditions under which people will stay well and enjoy the best quality of life that their community resources allow. In this way, the Ottawa Charter argues that health promotion is everyone's responsibility not just the individual's.

Of course, the emphasis on health and lifestyle has made health-promotion philosophy somewhat 'death-denying'. When people become seriously ill and encounter a life-threatening illness, health-promotion philosophy commonly falls silent. We 'slip-slop-slap' against the harmful effects of the sun's rays but when we are diagnosed with melanoma it is acute medical interventions that tend to be the total response to this calamity in a person's life. The social character of health, the notion of prevention and early intervention are ideals that seem to slip away and have little application for this situation. And yet there is no reason why these ideas should not be relevant.

The idea of health-promoting palliative care, however, is one that con-tinues to recognize the social character of living with life-threatening illness. Health-promoting palliative care recognizes issues about quality of life and the need for health maintenance even in the context of advanced disease. Being 'healthy' and experiencing 'disease', even 'terminal' disease, is not necessarily contradictory (Fryback 1993). The spiritual and social issues which strike at the heart of life-threatening illness can be addressed by health-promotion strategies – prevention, harm-reduction or early inter-vention – just as many of the physical and psychological issues can be addressed for these populations as they were in the early or middle years of their life and health.

Health-promoting palliative care is similar in its theory to health promo-tion in general. The goals of health-promoting palliative care are to provide education, information and policy-making for health, dying and death. It is incumbent upon health promotion when working with people with life-threatening illnesses to provide supports, both personal and community. It is important to encourage interpersonal reorientation. These changes in lifestyle may take in issues of sexual activity for example. These might range from managing one's seroconversion status with other sexual partners who may not be HIV positive to women managing vaginal thrush in cancer (a problem for women undergoing cancer treatments).

Palliative care services may need to be reoriented to offer health-promotion services. We have two problems here. Many palliative care services see their offerings in terms of face-to-face care at the end of life and not as services offering early intervention, as in community development. Research, policy development or post-diagnostic support and education groups may seem foreign, or to tax existing personnel and financial resources. Health promotion or community health services might see their mission in terms of targeting healthy populations so that they stay that way for as long as possible. Both kinds of service vision and activities need reorientation.

We should not lose health-promotion interest in anyone who has a life-threatening illness; witness the pioneering work with people living with HIV/AIDS. In the same way, palliative care was originally conceived as care of the dying post-diagnosis and across the course of the illness, not merely care in the last weeks of life. Neither Cicely Saunders nor the WHO originally conceived of hospice and palliative care in simple bedside terms. The funding priorities of government have frequently defined palliative care backwards, i.e. from the point of death rather than from the point of diagnosis. Health-promoting palliative care restores the priority of palliative care to its rightful place as a care that begins at diagnosis.

Finally, a health-promoting palliative care approach combats death-denying health policies and attitudes. Although health-promotion practices do exist with populations with life-threatening illness, in nearly every case these practices remove the problem of death and dying from their education and information resources. And yet, death education – from a personal examination of the fear of death to an exploration of what death means – is important to the control and management of fears in individuals, communities and professionals.

The task of 'making sense' of life at the end of life is an important task for those whose experience and expertise lies in health promotion and palliative care. The social and spiritual task and challenge of living life in the face of death should be a shared health-promotion task because its social significance applies to all of us, and because its successful management may be important to alleviating personal and physical pain.

In practice, the philosophy and theory of health promotion in palliative care takes on a variety of service forms, emanating as they do from clinical services in palliative care but also in more 'non-cancer' services, such as those for motor neuron disease. (The full range of practice suggestions for health-promoting palliative care have been described by Kellehear et al (2003).) Most of these involve the formation of adult learning groups led by people living with a life-threatening illness or a professional support worker. These groups are study and discussion groups that facilitate learning about their own health, life changes and death and dying.

Other health-promotion offerings by Australian palliative care services have included death education. This can and has included education about the history, sociology, psychology and spiritual understandings about death, dying, loss and the burden of care, and has been offered as patient and in-service staff education as well as community or public education programmes. Clinical services staff with an interest or talents in communicating with the general public have been encouraged to write about these experiences in the local press, to participate in talk-back radio or provide visits and talks to schools.

Other evidence of health-promotion activities in palliative care services has been expressed in the formation of partnerships with health-promotion or public health associations. These associations encourage palliative care staff, in their journal clubs or conference attendance for examples, to think about their service offerings in broader public health terms. The development of libraries that contain major holdings on the social and spiritual aspects of living with a life-threatening illness have also been important health-promotion offerings. Other holdings may cover experiences of death and loss, the sociology and history of death, and balanced and informative literature on alternative treatments. The library can be offered as a community resource, and not just something for dying people and their families to use.

Research and policy development is encouraged. But the research is social research rather than simply health services research. The experiences of people at the centre of dying, caring and loss, and the social meaning and consequences of those experiences, are prioritized as research and writing topics. Active political lobbying for extra financial resources to expand community services – a community role that feels completely foreign to most health practitioners – is a difficult role for palliative care services to adopt. Nevertheless, lobbying can also take the form of petitioning local community health services to share an interest in dying, death and loss with fellow workers who want to know about health promotion.

Along with policy work, the effort to create health-promoting settings is important but less attractive to service providers. The importance of thinking AND helping to create work, school or church environments that are sensitive to end-of-life care issues is seriously challenging for us all. Notwithstanding the growing presence of public health ideas in health-promoting palliative care in Australia (Palliative Care Australia 2003), what are emerging as its conceptual and practice limitations?

Six years after its original international publication and practice development in Australia, several critical observations are already apparent. Firstly, although health-promoting palliative care is a gentle way of introducing public health ideas to palliative care its practical introduction occurs largely within a clinical health services context. This means that willing and interested staff are confronted with the often difficult, sometimes impossible challenge of finding time, personnel and funding for these new offerings. These barriers say nothing of the retraining and education needs of these staff to provide health-promotion offerings with any confidence.

Secondly, assuming the willingness, training, time and personnel, most of the health-promotion offerings that most resemble *services to* the community tend to be prioritized. Support groups and patient education, for examples, are structures and processes that are familiar to clinical staff, so these gain attention quickly while broader community tasks tend to be neglected. Partnerships with other public or community health workers, the time needed to work with schools or municipal councils to create festivals of remembrance for example, take a low priority. Other services need significant time and funding resources to retrain volunteers to reorient to community development activities rather than bedside activities or home visits.

Thirdly, the rationalization for these activities to senior staff, medical staff or even to funding bodies can be difficult, complex and philosophically challenging. Interested staff can be, and have been, the subject of dismissive attitudes and professional challenge. The reformism and idealism that was so much a part of hospice history in the last 30 years seems now to have given way to a disturbing self-congratulatory attitude, a view that palliative care has the 'basics' right and is now 'consolidating' as a *'clinical speciality'* (Clark 2000: 54 (my emphasis)). Common instances of this resistance to new ideas in end-of-life care can pose significant barriers to viewing the field of palliative care as potential leaders in any vision or model of end-of-life care that might be viewed more broadly than simply bedside care of the terminally ill.

Fourthly, a health-promoting palliative care approach places much of the responsibility for initiating a public health approach to end-of-life care on palliative care services alone. This has two problems: end-of-life care is more than palliative care. Aged care, people living with loss from other sources of death and dying, the problem of suicide and other sudden death are not included in palliative care, yet these are relevant end-of-life care matters and experiences. And the placing of *all* the responsibility to *initiate* end-of-life care on palliative care is unfair and unrealistic. And to make matters worse, the field of public health itself seems slow to take up the challenge of work in end-of-life care.

Although palliative care might be expected to provide some leadership in this area, particularly with respect to the experience of terminal illness, there are other players in the health sector and beyond that must assume some major responsibility. It is vital that governments, for example, provide some policy leadership in the development and practice imperatives around public health approaches to dying, death and loss, if only to coordinate and maximize diverse service and community responses to death.

Finally, health promotion is only one public health approach but it tends to express itself in micropolitical terms. Education is a core component of all health promotion and this function makes it attractive to small group and small setting work, e.g. schools, nursing homes, workplaces, hospices and so on.

In this practical way, health promotion is user-friendly. It is easier to imagine and execute by small organizations and small groups of interested people. National governments are left to initiate and fund the larger ideas and projects, e.g. advertising programmes, sponsorship of festivals or school education programmes. *Institutional* mechanisms of social change that support health-promotion campaigns are frequently seen as beyond the ordinary and more modest capacity of services. And although behavioural change can and does lead to other social changes, other changes in law, municipal intervention or media policy can also create and complement equally valuable changes, however imposing, difficult or intimidating they might seem to initiate.

In these ways, health promotion is more available to conservative use and interpretation by those who would place the responsibility for change on individuals rather than communities or governments. But as the social history of medicine has revealed in the last chapter, only when governments are encouraged to think about health and death are these experiences changed in major, positive ways.

The idea that the major institutions of a society must change if there is to be an overall, sustainable improvement for the socially marginal or ill-affected by society is not new. Radical ideas for community change, even national change, have been articulated, debated and, to some extent, already taken up by others in many other health areas. We see these kinds of structural political suggestions in the recent history of psychiatry and disability and the normalization ideas of Wolfensberger (1975, 1992).

Can the ideas of normalization developed by Wolfensberger (1975, 1992) and supporters offer us a practical alternative to those of public health? Is normalization too radical a programme to expect, even to want, for a vision of end-of-life care? Can a public health approach achieve much the same goals for end-of-life care anyway?

Normalization theory

According to Emerson (1992), normalization is a family of ideas that began in Scandinavia with the work of Bank-Mikkelsen (1980) and Nirje (1970). They were some of the first writers to articulate the progressive view that the community has an obligation to reproduce the life of non-disabled people for disabled people. Government had a responsibility to integrate people with disabilities by creating communities that were user-friendly to the widest number and social type of people.

In the USA, Wolfensberger took these ideas further. Not content with simply 'mainstreaming' services and lifestyles for the disabled, Wolfensberger argued for the need to positively value people with disabilities. Communities need to create and support valued social roles for these people. We should overcompensate to combat their negative devalued positions. He called this set of more radical suggestions 'social role valorization' (Wolfensberger 1992). In the UK, John O'Brien embraced the Wolfensberger model and created from its general theory and assumptions a participatory model of service provision and use.

Although Wolfensberger's early work concerned services and social relations around people with disabilities, his later work was concerned with the problem of socially devalued people and roles in general. He believes that people are systematically devalued in a complex process that begins with their social labelling by others. A difference is selected out by others and a negative set of stories, attributes and deficiencies attached to this difference. Interestingly, a key stereotype used to dismiss the value of some people is to view them as dead or dying:

'The nearly dead, as good as dead, or already dead role is apt to be imposed on a seriously chronically ill person, a dying person, an aged person, and sometimes a disliked person, one condemned to death, or one who is seen as having "outlived usefulness"'

(Wolfensberger 1992: 12)

The stereotype of dying is just one of nine social labels of devaluation employed by communities to devalue others. In a society that has narrow and rigid normative criteria for power, success and inclusion, other labels employed to discredit others include: disabled, diseased, menacing, ridiculous, pitiful, poor, non-human and childlike.

The role of social role valorization is to create a set of social strategies that might literally reverse the fortunes of devalued people. The importance of employing these strategies revolves around social justice arguments – arguments about the need to address the negative social, psychological, physical and economic consequences to devalued people of their own marginality. People are rarely implicated in the creation of their differences, e.g. disability, gender or race. Rather, it is the social and cultural reaction to difference that is responsible for discrimination and unjust treatment.

Social role valorization targets seven areas of change in society. First, there must be consciousness-raising about the hidden assumptions that valued people make in relation to those marginalized. Secondly, there needs to be consciousness-raising about the sociology of deviance, in other words, an understanding about the way people react to each other as a consequence of labelling.

Thirdly, we must critically attack what Wolfensberger has called the 'conservatism corollary'. This means awareness about the social principle that eccentricity or deviant behaviour by people who are already regarded as deviant will be viewed more negatively than when others display the same behaviours. Affirmative action into positive roles is the only way to balance and correct this problem.

Fourthly, there must be a competence-enhancement programme that assumes all people can learn. Part of the problem with undesired and marginal groups is that they fail to understand how to 'pass'. Passing means a basic understanding about which unnecessary features in their behaviour or attitudes are creating barriers from others. Fifthly, the development of competence enhancement must include an understanding of the power and value of imitation and training.

The last two strategies include the importance of challenging and resisting cultural stereotypes, and the political and social push for integration of devalued types and their services. Communities must create and support recreational, workplace and educational policies of inclusion. Devalued people must be mainstreamed. Special clinical services for these people, if these are necessary, should not be in special designated areas but should be at sites where other services or other valued activities occur.

In the early twenty-first century we can easily see how these early 1970s ideas appeared radical, critical or unrealistic. And yet, many of these ideas have come to be integrated in the last quarter of a century in one way or another: in deinstitutionalization movements in psychiatry and disability; in the desire to make hospices and birthing centres 'home-like'; or in the placement of sheltered workshops or drug rehabilitation sites in middle-class suburbs.

We can see how some of these ideas played a role, if even a background one, in the early hospice and palliative care movements in Britain and the USA. Dying was a devalued, even denied, social role in hospitals during much of the twentieth century. Death represented medical failure and dying was the target of social stigma, rejection and embarrassment.

Few would disagree that the hospice movement worldwide has been a critical voice and a major challenge to these stereotypes, devalued experiences and hidden assumptions. There has been major consciousness-raising around our hidden professional and lay assumptions about dying, particularly in professional education. There has been major medical and nursing reform around the special care needs of dying people and their families. And for a while, hospice took dying people outside the traditional medical setting – the hospital – and rehabilitated the broad medical commitment to the patient to include the patient-as-dying person. But although some of the assumptions and reform strategy within hospice has overlapped with normalization ideas it is important to note where the similarities stop.

The recognition that the longer part of dying occurs outside of institutional settings and services has not been adequately addressed. Hospice and palliative care continue to see the problem-based aspects of dying without identifying a positive community role for themselves around normal aspects of living with a life-threatening illness. There has been little to no attempt to challenge cultural stereotypes about dying. Few, if any, connections are made between cancer death and other forms of death and dying. The grief of bereavement has not been connected with other sources of grief in the community. White people's loss, for example, has not been connected with black people's loss.

The influence of normalization in palliative care, such as it is, has been confined to institutional understandings about services and professional relationships, and not the relationships between dying, loss and community identity and context. Community is a background idea in palliative care, not a foreground issue. The field of palliative care defines its role in clinical terms of palliation, repair and support, not as a public educator, community member or policy leader. The patient and family are the objects of care, not the community and nation. In these ways, normalization is a tempering rather than shaping influence on the field of palliative care.

There has been criticism of normalization (see Emerson 1992). Some have argued that normalization has merely moved us from a treatment model to an advocacy one. Professionals remain the people most interested in these matters, not the disabled or psychiatrically impaired people so much at the centre of these theories (Whitehead 1992). Many of the changes have had little evaluation to establish their objective value (McGill and Emerson 1992). Normalization also creates a reified idea of the 'normal', ignoring that communities and societies are pluralist, representing diverse populations and interests (Dalley 1992). There is also insufficient recognition that there are limits to integration and 'mainstreaming' (Szivos 1992). And integration may not even be desired, or of value, by and to the very groups that normalization claims to champion (Brown and Smith 1992).

Much of this criticism is valid, but the devil is in the detail and not the overall policy direction and suggestions of the theory. And it is the broad policy assumptions and suggestions that have been taken up in reforms across most of the industrial world in the last 30 years. Normalization theory highlights the widespread problem that many people have with social and physical differences of others. It highlights the social justice issues that stem from that problem.

The policy suggestions of normalization encourage positive changes in professional identity. We should not think it a small achievement to have moved professional responses from treatment to advocacy positions. This is an important move from a paternalistic approach to human services to one more closely resembling a partnership. It is true that not all devalued people desire integration, or not all of the time or not with just anyone in the community. The recognition of valued social and cultural networks and affinities is important to a critical understanding of 'integration'. But without the advocacy of integration the individual and policy space to make a choice of this kind is not there at all. And the choice of social site must surely be part of a sophisticated and caring response to social services of any kind.

Normalization theory then is primarily a theory of social justice that highlights the personal and political consequences of social inequality. It draws our attention to the social processes that are responsible for these conditions and that can be changed by us. The proponents and critics of normalization at least agree that those changes can only be brought about not by a continuation of traditional clinical services but rather by taking a *social* approach to the problem. In so far as normalization changes bring about improvements to the health and quality of life of those devalued, normalization approaches are public health ones. They strike at the heart of the need for coordinated changes in several social institutions, not just those in health or social services. But in the matter of end-of-life care, normalization does not go far enough.

End-of-life care is not fully addressed by debating place of death, site of service or the integration of ageing and dying people in the community, no matter how worthwhile these issues obviously are. Nor is end-of-life care simply a problem of 'valorizing' or strengthening the perceived value of undesirable roles such as terminally ill, old person or suicide survivor, although once again these are important tasks to perform. This is because normalization theory and strategies are theories and strategies of *rehabilitation for some*. It is an approach designed to correct wrongs and to analyse and tackle the problem – perceived or actual – of social abnormality.

On the other hand, public health is a theory and set of action strategies designed to enhance *the health and well-being of all*. Although that aim may include theories of repair and social correction, this is only *part* of the scientific and community efforts to raise awareness of how communities can strengthen their usual cultural and social capital to maximize their own health and well-being.

For a public health approach to end-of-life care this means not only understanding and addressing devalued roles such as ageing and dying but also the *universal and normative* experiences of death, loss and grief. Public health approaches to end-of-life care must address dying, death loss and care as normal and usual experiences for which communities can and should take some responsibility.

Towards a public health approach to end-of-life care

Psychosocial palliative care has inadequate concepts and strategies to deal with community building and partnership tasks associated with public health practices. The commitment to a 'bedside' palliative care practice – a practice understood in treatment intervention terms – has meant that in training and occupational profile, palliative care comes ill-equipped for the challenge of public health end-of-life care.

Health-promoting palliative care ideas tend to attract attention mainly in areas or topics that favour a direct-services type approach. Community building or policy development topics and activities attract far less attention by practitioners, again partly because of the training and occupational deficits in this field. In simple theoretical terms, health-promoting palliative care is able to provide a basis for a broader public health approach if the training and occupational profile of current palliative care practitioners was broadened.

Normalization theories are strong on community and policy development but have the major disadvantage of placing all their attention on devalued roles, marginal social experiences and the general problem of social inequality. In these ways, normalization approaches are both too narrow to encompass universal human experiences and, because of that fact, are conceptually deficient in supplying strategies to address universal and normative experiences. Additionally, most of the descriptive policy suggestions tend to concentrate around the problem of disabilities with end-of-life care offered minimal practice suggestion. This, of course, is a historical artefact of the early interest that normalization theorists had in disability.

An adequate public health approach to end-of-life care must make central to its strategies, concepts that are health promoting, community building and partnership oriented. Strategies that derive from these concepts must stress the traditional public health practices of prevention, policy development, government leadership and intersectorial cooperation. The approach that best meets these criteria is one based on the WHO idea of the Healthy City. I have called this Healthy City version of communities that care for each other at the end-of-life 'Compassionate Cities'.

Chapter 3

Theoretical foundations of Compassionate Cities

The idea of the Compassionate City is derived from a global public health approach to the promotion of community-wide strategies for health entitled 'Healthy Cities'. The Healthy Cities projects were developed by the World Health Organization (WHO) as one way to implement the Ottawa Charter for Health Promotion (1986). Action strategies are designed for the health of whole communities across a diverse range of its sectors – workplaces, recreational sites and events, schools and universities, nursing homes and hospitals and in churches, local government and voluntary organizations.

This intersectorial approach to public health draws heavily on the idea that the personal experience of health depends on strong and sustainable social foundations – partnerships, community involvement and supports, reorientation of health services and the development of personal skills for all citizens. The premier assumption of this public health approach is that health is not merely the absence of disease. In a parallel way, quality of life is not merely the absence of problems.

But notwithstanding these worthy ideas about health and quality of life, the experience of death, dying and loss is largely absent from the language, theory and policy direction of Healthy Cities. Ironically, the earlier idea of death as failure, so characteristic of medical thinking in the middle of the twentieth century, seems to suggest itself in current health-promotion theory and policy (Kellehear 1999a: 14–15). In this chapter I want to trace the theoretical foundations for a public health model of end-of-life care that is inclusive of the experiences of dying, death and loss. I will outline the basic theoretical assumptions and concepts of the Compassionate City by modifying and extending the current theory and concepts of Healthy Cities.

First, I will introduce readers to the definition, history and central concepts of Healthy Cities. I will then define Compassionate Cities in terms of their theoretical and policy similarities to Healthy Cities. A conceptual comparison between a psychosocial approach to palliative care and this Compassionate City approach will be discussed. Finally, I will examine the major criticism and objections to the idea of large-scale, sociological models of health and end-of-life care. I will ask and reply to questions about their practicality, relevance, relative success, and value to current goals of public health and palliative care.

Introduction to Healthy Cities

According to Ashston et al (1986) the very origins of public health can be traced to its health-promotion initiatives developed in eighteenth and nineteenth century cities. The squalor, undernourishment and infectious diseases so responsible for the mortality and morbidity of those periods led directly to the establishment of municipal public health departments. The growing disillusionment with the costs and effectiveness of direct medical services and the therapeutics industry of today has led to a recent revival of interest in public health ideas.

The psychiatrist and public health worker Leonard Dahl (Aicher 1998) had contributed writings that examined and developed ideas towards holistic and systemic approaches to health. In 1984 a major public health conference was held in Toronto, Canada, to explore ecological and holistic approaches to health policy and it was at this forum that Dahl coined the phrase 'Healthy Cities' (Aicher 1998: xii).

Taking the view that health was a quality of life inexorably linked to 'habitats' – to the immediate, physical and social environments of organisms including human organisms – seemed like a good idea. In particular, this was viewed well given the likelihood that by 2000 almost half the world's population would live in cities. The idea of the city as a primary site for strategic health policy approaches also seemed appropriate: cities are the most basic political and administrative level for assembling political and financial resources, and engaging participation and intersectorial cooperation.

From this academic and policy pressure to view health in these wider and more interdependent relationships, several other initiatives were developed and/or coincided. In 1986, the WHO published the Ottawa Charter for Health Promotion. This consisted of five important principles for the environmental support of health. These principles were: building healthy public policies; creating supportive environments; developing community action; developing personal skills; and the reorientation of health services. In that same year (1986), the Lisbon Symposium on Healthy Cities took place with participants from 21 cities. Drawing from the WHO policy statements on 'Health for All' and the 'Ottawa Charter', this conference began to establish some of the first definitions and action statements around the idea of Healthy Cities. In 1987 Healthy Cities was established as an actual policy programme of WHO's European Regional Office (Baum 1998: 445).

Since these beginnings, Healthy Cities programmes have been established worldwide. By 1992 the WHO office worked directly with 35 cities.

The 20-step booklet that outlines the initial steps for the establishment of a Healthy City programme has been translated into over 20 languages. Since 1995, Healthy Cities programmes have extended into Eastern and Central Europe and Asia, with cities cooperating with each other on specific health-promotion campaigns (Tsouros 1995).

What is a Healthy City? According to Hancock and Dahl (1985) and Tsouros (1990: 20), a Healthy City has 11 qualities that it should strive toward. Healthy Cities should be clean, safe environments. They have an ecosystem that is stable now and sustainable in the long term. Healthy Cities are characterized by strong mutually supportive environments, and have high degrees of community participation and control over decisions that affect their lives. The basic needs of food and shelter are being met in these cities. There is access to a wide variety of positive experiences and resources, and a diverse and innovative economy. Healthy Cities encourage connectedness with the spiritual and cultural traditions of the past as well as with other diverse groups within the community. The social and physical forms – key organizations and events in the community – actually enhance these above-mentioned qualities. Finally, there should be an optimum level of health and welfare services that are accessible to all, and a high health status in the general population, i.e. high levels of health and low levels of disease. The WHO summarized these characteristics of Healthy Cities into nine principles (WHO 1996: 15).

Box 1 World Health Organization definition of a Healthy City

- Has a clean, safe physical environment
- Meets the basic needs of all its inhabitants
- Has a strong mutually supportive, integrated non-exploitative community
- Involves community in local government
- Offers inhabitants access to wide variety of experiences, interactions and communications
- Promotes and celebrates its historical and cultural heritage
- Provides easily accessible health services
- Has a diverse, innovative economy
- Rests on a sustainable ecosystem

The three underlying concepts of the Healthy City then are: (1) health is a positive concept, it is not simply the absence of disease; (2) health is a holistic concept – in other words, the establishment and maintenance of good health depends on the nurturing role of the physical, social, political, economic and spiritual environment, not simply the quality of direct health services alone, i.e. health is an ecological idea, not a medical one; finally (3), Healthy Cities must always be concerned with inequalities in health – health, like wealth, is unevenly distributed in the population and any genuine concern about health must address the differential way in which health distributes itself among those of different ages, genders, ethnicity and social classes (Hancock 1993).

Box 2 Central concepts of Healthy Cities

- Health is a positive concept
- Health is a holistic/ecological idea
- Health is a concern for inequalities in health

(Hancock 1993)

How are such broad ideas to be translated into practical action? There has been much written about the translation, implementation and evaluation of these broad policy ideas. The WHO's 20 steps in developing a Healthy Cities project will be discussed in the later practice chapters of this book but, for the moment, I have found little that does not conform to the simple prescriptions of Ashton et al (1986). Although WHO's steps cover theory preparation, organization and evaluation, Ashton et al (1986) simply cover what to do in that first year of setting up.

First, one should establish an intersectorial Healthy Cities Committee as a decision-making committee of the city council. An Implementation Group who will be steered/guided into action will represent a subcommittee of the decision-making committee. One should also explore the possibility of establishing a 'Health Ombudsman' to develop and complement the advocacy functions of the municipality. There should be some evidence that a public debate about the creation of a Healthy City has occurred. There should be a minimal data set about the current health of the community. This should include health-enhancing activities of the community as well as morbidity data. There should be a population survey of at least two population subgroups, e.g. immigrants, women or the unemployed. There should be partnerships with local research institutions such as universities to establish a set of research questions to assist in the development and evaluation of the community's health. There should be a demonstrated working relationship with the media. There should be a review of current health-promotion activities in the city. There should be a forum of non-government organizations involved with health to tackle a specific health issue. There should also be cooperation with local museums, art galleries, theatres and schools to help create and support education about health. And finally, there needs to be active working links with other Healthy City projects for the purposes of information exchange and support.

Box 3 Making Healthy Cities happen

- Create a steering and implementation committee at city hall
- Create and document public debate about Healthy Cities
- Research the city's current health and illness profile
- Pay particular attention to current health inequalities in the city
- Work with the local media
- Cooperate with local cultural institutions
- Support local health education initiatives
- Create partnerships with non-government sectors
- Exchange information and experience with other Healthy Cities

(From Ashton et al (1986))

This definition and these concepts that support Healthy Cities are also the theoretical foundations for the idea of Compassionate Cities, for no theory of public health can ignore the universal problem of death, disability and loss. And no theory of a Compassionate City can be built without assuming that, in the first place, that city is a Healthy City. In other words, just as health and quality of life are experiences founded on ecological relationships to social, physical and political support systems, so too the idea of compassion must be viewed as an idea and experience founded on the principle of social interdependencies.

Introduction to Compassionate Cities

The word 'compassion' means to pity or to share or show mercy and sympathy in another person's suffering. The term 'compassionate' is to have this quality of attitude and action. It is a commiseration – a joint journey of sharing with another. Funk and Wagnell's *New Standard Dictionary of the English Language* (Funk 1963) observes that the term 'compassion' derives from two Latin root words: 'cum' meaning 'together' and 'patior' meaning 'suffer'.

But under the terms 'compassion, compassionate', Partridge's (1958: 113) *Dictionary of Etymology* provides the intriguing advice 'See patience'. Under this term, we learn that Latin prefix-compounds such as 'pati', that are root origins for compassion and compassionate, are Old French terms adopted from Late Latin. This root suggests a *sharing with* another's suffering; to be patient in another's suffering, to bear and support suffering. This 'pati' root also has another etymological life as the basis for the

English term 'patient' – a person who shows patience, presumably in his or her own suffering.

In policy and etymological senses it is important to emphasize this focus on mutual sharing. This idea is quite different from our ideas about *caring*. The term 'care' derives from the Old English terms 'carean', 'cearu' and 'caru', meaning grief and sorrow and is akin to the Old Saxon word 'kara' – a lament (Partridge 1958: 79–80). So the verb to 'care' is to grieve, be troubled or to take thought for another (Onion 1966: 145–6). According to *The Barnhart Dictionary of Etymology* (Barnhart 1988: 144), 'The word is cognate, in the primary sense of inward grief . . .' and not connected with the Latin 'cura' (care) '. . . in the sense of pains and troubles bestowed on others'. I need to add here that the sociological implication of this particular meaning of 'care' as 'cure' has led to an unequal understanding of helping that involves the well helping the sick, the 'professional' helping the lay, the knowledgeable one assisting the one who knows not. Sociologically speaking, this is precisely what 'compassion' is not. Death and loss belong to all of us in small and big ways, sooner or later, in a literal embodied sense or symbolically and psycho-dynamically. Compassionate approaches are partnership approaches literally, sociologically and in policy meanings. They are the foundations of social empathy.

The idea of the Compassionate City is not entirely new for it can trace its history to at least Europe in the Middle Ages. For example, Sennett (1994) describes a crucial time in the development of Western cities when 'compassion' developed as an important topic of medicine, politics and social policy. The Middle Ages witnessed a rising tension between church, state and economy, a time when the rise of dispassionate mercantile values seemed to conflict with the very human basis of religion and society itself – the need for human beings to treat each other with empathy, fairness and kindness.

In other words, the development of the modern city in the Middle Ages created a social tension between the need to establish new relationships free of traditional obligations, so that one could buy and sell without social bias, and the ongoing need to develop caring relationships. A society-wide conversation arose, a discourse that remains equally relevant today, that attempted to reforge the modern citizen's responsibilities in commerce with those of their parallel responsibilities toward each other as vulnerable fellow human beings, i.e. as compassionate people (Sennett 1994: 159).

Sennett (1994) described a number of religious and medical discourses of the times that attempted to promote and assert the 'naturalness' of compassion. The parallels between Christ's suffering during the crucifixion and our own and other's daily suffering reminded caring people that their social feelings were an imitation of the religious feeling about Jesus on the cross. In the medical observations and theories about sympathetic bodily reactions to injuries and disease – how heat and blood flow would move from healthy organs to injured ones – these mimicked the compassion of the holy for the sinful. Compassion and altruism had a basis in nature as well as the soul. The body in these storylines became metaphors, even prescriptions, for the medieval city as a Compassionate City. We are beginning to witness a return to this kind of Compassionate City in the early writings and experiments of public health.

But the theoretical as opposed to the historical reasons for the choice of the term 'compassionate' is to signal a number of ethical and policy distinctions that the current term 'health' does not seem to make in the current public health/health-promotion discourse. These are first, that compassion is an ethical imperative for health. Compassion is the human response, the tender response aroused by the distress and suffering of others. It is the moral, social, political and physical basis of our attempts to give aid and support in a time of difficulty. A healthy person without compassion is a potentially dangerous person to the health and safety of other people.

Second, health is a positive concept that can coexist in the presence of disease, disability or loss. WHO stress that health is not simply the absence of disease. On the contrary, for most of us disease is ever present. No conception of health makes sense without acknowledgement that, to more or less extent, diseases such as atherosclerosis, arthritis, hypertension, diabetes and many other diseases singly or together affect most of the population. Disabilities in movement, sight, hearing or touch are endemic. Indeed, chronic illness and disability are so widespread that any definition of health that excludes these experiences promotes an unnecessarily idealistic, in fact, unrealistic, idea of health. Disease is not the opposite of health, death is.

Third, compassion is a holistic/ecological concept just as much as are current public health conceptions of health. Compassion must express itself not simply in an individual attitude but in changes in the workplace, churches, human services and schools. Death and loss must be recognized as universal experiences that we all share, and provision for these experiences must be integrated in policies and practices at those sites.

Finally, compassion necessarily implies a concern with the universality of loss. Loss can result from terminal illness (cancer, AIDS, motor neuron disease, etc.) but also violence (victims of crime and abuse). The forced separation of peoples from their land or their cultural traditions and identity (refugees, indigenous peoples and international adoptions) must make dispossession equal to bereavement as a compassionate concern for end-of-life care. This pivots our attention from the meaning of the term 'end' in this phrase, as a biographical and physical end of 'an individual life' to a wider understanding of loss and identity as connections and endings to a broader community life within and outside ourselves.

In this above context, of course, social and physical rejection (from racism, sexism, ageism, disability, relationship disintegration or unemployment) is equally a concern, not only because these concern all Healthy Cities as issues of inequality but also as compassionate issues. They are compassionate issues because they create death and loss in others in their social, symbolic and sometimes even physical lives. They are 'risk' factors in the identification and control of dispassionate ('heartless') attitudes, values and policies by individuals and governments. They are legitimate concerns of a Compassionate City approach to public health policy and practice.

Box 4 Central concepts of Compassionate Cities

- Compassion is an ethical imperative for health
- Health is a positive concept even in the presence of disease, disability or loss
- Compassion is a holistic/ecological idea
- Compassion implies a concern with the universality of loss

How do these central concepts of the Compassionate City translate into defining characteristics? There are nine characteristics that define a Compassionate City and these should be read together with the nine WHO defining characteristics of Healthy Cites. These are: Compassionate Cities have local health policies that recognize compassion as an ethical imperative. There must be a public debate about the value and need for compassion to be an ethical imperative in their environments, and for health to take up the hard challenge of genuinely viewing health away from physical experience. We must make and debate the practical links between ethical choices and supportive health-promoting environments.

Compassionate Cities also meet the special needs of its aged, those living with life-threatening illness and those living with loss. There must be new connections forged between experiences of mortality, health and quality of life that are now frequently viewed as counter-intuitive. There can and should be an acknowledgement that death and loss are predictable and permanent experiences, and that we can and should strive for quality of life rather than denial in their shadow. Compassionate Cities, as Healthy Cities, also have a strong commitment to social and cultural difference. There can be no safety and therefore no guarantees for health in a community that does not passionately advocate tolerance and embrace difference. While we live in a time and a place where only some people are viewed as deserving of all the rights and privileges of community support, no one is safe.

Compassionate Cities also involve the grief and palliative care services in local government policy and planning. No planning, policy development or set of action strategies can be designed or implemented without the experience and insights of those who have made a professional life studying and caring for those facing death and loss. Compassionate Cities must also offer their inhabitants access to a wide variety of supportive experiences, interactions and communication. Unless people who face death and loss are able to see themselves, see their own experiences reflected in the face of their own community, in the local media, then marginalization, alienation and despair will always be unshared, private experiences.

Compassionate Cities also promote and celebrate reconciliation with indigenous peoples and the memory of other important community losses. We will not understand the cultural and existential basis for loss while we continue to see this experience in the narrow and confined terms of bereavement. Death and loss have a wider meaning beyond disease, and these experiences and consequences need to be recognized and understood to create inclusive policies on loss that mean the most to most people.

Compassionate Cities also provide easy access to grief and palliative care services. Because many of these services are historically new, they play a major role in current support of people facing death and loss, and have created a cutting-edge body of knowledge for those of us in public health who would take end-of-life care forward and beyond those services. Compassionate Cities also recognize and plan to accommodate those disadvantaged by the economy, including rural and remote populations, indigenous people and the homeless. In these ways again, Compassionate Cities as Healthy Cities concern themselves with inequalities.

Finally, a Compassionate City preserves and promotes a community's spiritual traditions and storytellers. Beyond mere social and health beliefs, the spiritual traditions of a community – particularly its religions and cosmic belief systems – are a treasury of ideas about death, suffering and loss, and will be instrumental in the provision of support and comfort. Compassionate Cities are not only mindful of public health ideas, they are respectful and supportive of diverse religious beliefs, its direction, desire and, when relevant, its absence.

Box 5 Defining characteristics of a Compassionate City

- Has local health policies that recognize compassion as an ethical imperative
- Meets the special needs of its aged, those living with life-threatening illness and those living with loss
- Has a strong commitment to social and cultural difference
- Involves the grief and palliative care services in local government policy and planning
- Offers its inhabitants access to a wide variety of supportive experiences, interactions and communication
- Promotes and celebrates reconciliation with indigenous peoples and the memory of other important community losses
- Provides easy access to grief and palliative care services
- Has a recognition of and plans to accommodate those disadvantaged by the economy, including rural and remote populations, indigenous people and the homeless
- Preserves and promotes a community's spiritual traditions and storytellers

---

The above definitions and theoretical characteristics of Healthy and Compassionate Cities highlight a major departure from current ways of thinking about end-of-life care, particularly palliative care. The current interpretation of palliative care as clinical care at the end-of-life is not community care, however appropriate and worthy in its own medical terms. In other words, contemporary palliative care draws on a tradition of concepts that currently creates barriers toward taking a leadership role in any public health approach to end-of-life care such as that outlined for Compassionate Cities.

I will now compare and contrast the sociological assumptions of palliative care with those of public health to identify the reasons why a Compassionate City approach can, but may not easily, emanate from current interests within palliative care. There are several major challenges and limits to the current practice wisdom and vision of palliative care. On the one hand, there are other more outward-looking assumptions within palliative care that seem to make it conceptually suitable to extending its work beyond institutional settings. However, palliative medical interests in particular seem to shy away from public health ideas of any kind, and this source of conservatism within palliative care may lead to resistance and barriers to implementation of compassionate policies and priorities.

Continuities and difficulties for palliative care

There are seven conceptual tensions between the ideas of palliative care and those underlying public health. The size and significance of the future role that palliative care may play in the development of public health approaches to end-of-life care will, to a very significant extent, depend on how successful these tensions are negotiated internally to that field.

First, palliative care is patient-centred. The needs of patients are primary in the development of all care plans. Wherever possible, it is the service or the hospice that must attempt to adjust and adapt to the wishes and autonomy of the patient and his or her social and personal choices. This patient-centred approach is a major historical departure from a profession-centred approach where the desires of professionals and the routines of hospitals have prevailed, and still prevail, in many institutional settings.

Patienthood versus citizenship

Nevertheless, a patient-centred approach, however admirable and crucial this idea might be in institutional settings, will not be adequate nor workable in a public health scenario. Public health simply does not have 'patients'. Public health approaches to health, such as Compassionate Cities, assume people are free citizens, not patients in some sort of custodial relationship with a health care provider.

Citizenship recognizes that people in modern society have a set of civil, political and social reciprocities with the key institutions within their society. These are mutual obligations between governments and laws, employers and employees, families and churches, and even to each other as mere strangers passing each other on the street. Citizenship is the key way that modern societies attempt to mediate the inequalities imposed differentially upon them by the vagaries of market economies, gender and ethnic inequalities, and the serendipity of acquired or inherited social status (Turner 1993).

The Western notion of citizenship is closely bound up with membership of modern nation states and particularly cities. Thus, 'The French term "citoyen" is derived from "cite", which refers to an assembly of citizens who enjoy certain limited rights within a city' (Turner 1993: 9). Citizenship creates social solidarity despite social differences, but in so doing can create potential conflicts over entitlements. The citizen is socially, politically and legally equal to all other citizens. In this framework and language, health becomes an entitlement and not simply a service. The role of palliative care is not service provision in this framework but community partner – a reciprocal partnership in education AND learning. Whether palliative care can transform its understanding from services and learning for patients to partnerships with citizens and learning from communities will depend on how well and how genuine the early patient-centred approach translates to a citizen-centred one.

Health services versus social capital

Palliative care is also a relative newcomer to the health system and there is a need to impress governments and the community of the need for greater funding. This is particularly important in two ways: for greater geographical coverage of these new services to all communities within the one country; and for greater professional development needs, i.e. to include a greater number of occupations within the multidisciplinary team. These professional concerns focus on building and strengthening the health service but, although these are important aims for palliative care as the newest member of that institution, these aims do not enhance or contribute to a public health approach such as Compassionate Cities.

A Compassionate City approach will require dedication to 'social capital'. Social capital is a relatively new phrase with a diversity of meanings and more than a little debate about their distinction with former understandings of human or physical capital (Fine 2001, Lin et al 2001). Nevertheless, there is broad agreement that the term social capital covers valued social activities such as cooperation for mutual benefit, community participation and support, levels of community trust and respect, and the degree to which communities interact with one another (Bourdieu 1980, Coleman 1988, Baum 1999).

Compassionate Cities create opportunities for community members to come together, establish networks, and develop trusting and caring relations with one another. Compassionate Cities, like Healthy Cities, create a policy space for building community solidarity, not from the addition of more health or social services but through rising levels of communication, respect and trust. Baum (1998: 94) cites the 1993 study by Putnam (1993) of why some Italian regional governments succeeded more than others did. He found that high levels of civic engagement, participation and solidarity were the most important differentiating factors responsible. Palliative care's ability to move away from an understandable self-interest over the consolidation of its health services empire, to make room for ideas and strategies that build social capital in a community, so that these communities are better able to support themselves in death and loss, will be a challenge.

Family versus community

Palliative care is not simply committed to patients, but patients and their families. The support network of patients, such as their friends and family, are important 'units' of care, and particularly after the patient has died, they may need bereavement support and/or follow up. Many palliative care services, if resources are available, are committed to providing this family support during the dying process and after the death of the patient. But family is not community, only a part of the community. It is one, albeit an important one, of several key institutions within a society.

To what extent can cities be said to be communities anymore? How easily can we embrace the romantic notion, even for rural towns and villages, that organizations such as these are 'genuine' communities? All social groupings have people who are regarded as insiders and outsiders. There are outcasts and deviants, people with multiple identities, both open and covert. There are lawbreakers and sociopaths in most communities, big or small. What is support for some is invasion for others.

Yet, recent studies of communities and how they work (or don't) show that the most important ties and supports that people successfully employ for themselves are based on simple networks. These may be in cities or rural areas. They can be suburban networks or ones based on kin. The important element involved in these networks is that people understand how to access and use them, how to communicate effectively within them, and the stability and support people gain from them. Terms such as 'community' or 'city' matter less than the idea that these networks are extensive and go well beyond the idea or realities of 'family'. The important function and advantage that employing the term 'community' has over 'family' is that the complexity of direct support is better captured by the former than by the latter.

Until now, palliative care has viewed 'community' as an abstract idea similar to the 'general public' and not as a set of specific networks that are capable of sharing the burden of care in practical ways beyond members of a family. Re-examining the meaning of community through a Compassionate City policy approach will allow palliative care to extend its understanding of ideas such as 'family' and 'community based' care by taking these ideas into workplaces, schools and trade union organizations. Only within these kinds of social contexts and networks will the idea of 'community based' transform into a genuine community development, a framework that not only extends the idea of family but underpins and supports it.

Palliative care holism versus public health holism

Palliative care is holistic care. This means that patient care is not simply care of the physical needs of the patient but also his or her social, psychological and spiritual needs. This has been a long-standing commitment of palliative care and has led to commitment to the next feature of palliative care. Public health has also been holistic care. But the meaning of holism to palliative care and public health has been dramatically different. Palliative care has employed the following language to describe this commitment: social, physical, psychological and spiritual. Public health, on the other hand, has employed different language to describe its understanding of holism: the nomenclature of ecology, politics, community, settings and environments.

So while the holistic approach of palliative care has emphasized the whole person as individual, public health has emphasized the whole person as individual-in-community. The person-as-individual is very much a function of providing services to persons as patients receiving that help in institutions such as hospices or hospitals or as patients at home. Here it is the individual AWAY from their obvious community context and connections that individuals are being seen. The 'whole person' care is disembodied care – the body and mind of the person is disconnected from his or her usual physical place at the work desk, the bar, the club, the church or the theatre. The whole person is really the whole patient.

The public health view of whole person is the whole person as citizen. It is the person at the club, theatre or work desk, and it is at those sites that Compassionate or Healthy Cities approaches must engage those persons in taking an interest in their own health or compassionate care. Although there is an undoubtedly genuine commitment to holistic care of the dying from palliative care, that idea of holism is yet to spread to include settings and environments and the politics of life as lived in the community. Even an understanding of the phrase 'whole person care' will need a significant shift to a settings understanding for palliative care to grasp the ecological challenge of Compassionate Cities.

Occupational versus community capacity building

Palliative care has been dedicated to occupational capacity building. Because dying is not a medical phenomenon but a human one, the needs of the dying person are multidimensional and therefore can only be adequately addressed by a multidisciplinary team approach. Palliative care agencies have always attempted to employ or be in partnerships with occupations such as social work, pastoral care or chaplaincy, and psychology as well as nursing and medicine.

Compassionate and Healthy Cities approaches to care require a commitment to community capacity building. Community capacity building can be performed 'top-down within', meaning leadership initiates changes to people below in organization. Or capacity building can be performed 'bottom-up within' by people at ground level to change organizational cultures. There can also be 'partnerships' by some organizations with others. There can also be attempts by members of the community to start new organizations. Either way, the aim of capacity building is to raise people's awareness of their own abilities, knowledge and skills that permit them to employ available support systems, problem solve, take decisions, and communicate and act more effectively.

Capacity building is about encouraging communities and organizations to reach their goals more effectively by using what they have more effectively (Crisp et al 2000). Again, this capacity building as a potential aim of palliative care services will require a reorientation of the usual service aims, particularly since it will involve community development rather than didactic educational functions by those services. It will also require a recognition that addressing complex human needs is not simply adding yet another occupation to the ever-growing 'interdisciplinary team'.

Palliative care versus palliative approach

Palliative care has also recognized that much can be done, and should be done, before the 'terminal', i.e. last phase, of life. Palliative care is not simply care of people in the last days or hours of life. There is also recognition and practice of the 'palliative approach', an approach that does not deal directly with the final time before death but provides health services well before that time to assist in the promotion and maintenance of a person's quality of life (Finlay and Jones 1995). Here, within the model of the palliative approach, lies a policy and practice space inside existing palliative care theory that would recognize and facilitate a public health approach to end-of-life care. Compassionate Cities are a palliative approach to quality of life and end-of-life care that recognize the need to employ early intervention strategies, both in the matter of social contexts and relationships.

Nevertheless, the theoretical recognition and the occupational realities are other matters altogether. The fact is that palliative care has an occupational profile best fitting an institutional model of care, i.e. doctors, nurses, social workers with casework interests and psychologists. The employment of community development workers – health educators, social workers specializing in community work, pastoral care workers who see their role as community members more than counsellors, all these occupations and epistemological assumptions are uncommon in contemporary palliative care. Although the palliative approach and commitment is present, the current occupational and funding infrastructure is wanting and may be insufficient to meet the challenge.

Cancer care versus end-of-life care

Finally, palliative care has largely dealt with cancer patients. This has been a historical artefact of the early work of Cicely Saunders, but people with this disease have been the major beneficiaries to date. It is true that some people living with AIDS and neurological diseases have also been cared for by palliative care services but these groups are in the minority overall.

The demography of death and dying however tells us a different picture of dying, and hence promises us a different picture of the future of palliative care. According to Lynn (2002), about 7% of Americans will die suddenly, about 22% of people will die of cancer, another 16% will die of cardiovascular system diseases such as strokes and cardiac failure, and about 45% of people will simply die of 'old age', by which is meant they will grow so old that their medical problems will be multiple. These aged people will be in various stages of cardiac, renal or liver failure; they may also have a diagnosed cancer. But no one of these disease states will necessarily cause their death. More likely, a mild respiratory infection will tip the balance for the worse in a bodily context of few-to-no reserves. For most of those who will die of cardiac problems and for the overwhelming number of old people who will pass their final days in nursing homes and hospitals, few will see a palliative care service.

Neither the symptoms of cardiac problems nor the multiple problems of the frail aged exempt them from palliative care, e.g. most will have the same or greater needs for the specialist skills of palliative medicine and nursing. However, the challenge of caring for these populations outside of institutional settings, of addressing their *social* care issues in non-clinical ways, are all challenges and skill gaps for contemporary palliative care, rehabilitation medicine and gerontology. There are limits to professional help in these kinds of end-of-life community scenarios. We have been slow to recognize these limits to professional care.

The distinction between end-of-life medical issues and end-of-life social issues are subtle. Care of frail elderly, and those whose physical deterioration is unpredictable, is a health issue for all of us who share a community life with those people. This is a broad public health problem and one that only equally broad community strategies and capabilities can address adequately. The questions are: will palliative care view its responsibilities as stopping at service provision, and will it enhance and support public health strategies that support a palliative approach to prevention and quality of life at the end-of-life?

Box 6   Conceptual tensions in palliative care and public health

- Patienthood versus citizenship
- Health services versus social capital
- Family versus community
- Palliative care holism versus public health holism
- Occupational capacity building versus community capacity building
- Palliative care versus palliative approach
- Cancer care versus end-of-life care

Compassionate Cities: criticism and response

There are a number of reoccurring criticisms of Healthy Cities and because of the theoretical kinship of Compassionate Cities these criticisms also apply to this more recent formulation. In general, we can identify four major criticisms of Healthy and Compassionate Cities. These are distinct from major threats to Compassionate Cities in anyone's attempt to establish and sustain an ongoing programme: I will address those problems in Chapter 6.

The criticism levelled at sociological approaches to public health such as Compassionate Cities is that the idea of a 'community' is largely a myth anyway. Secondly, those Healthy City type ideas are utopian ones with little practical value or reality. Third, that even Healthy Cities that currently exist are marginal to the main economic and health services work of promoting health, and interest in them is waning. Finally, Healthy Cities are too difficult to evaluate and this makes them unjustifiable in the current climate of fiscal restraint and high competition for scarce public resources.

Community: myth or reality

There has been much debate (for a review of some of this material see Mayo 1994, 2000), particularly in the social sciences, about whether this idea has any genuine cultural substance as an idea. Crow and Allan (1994) provide some practical arguments about why the idea still has merit. The first and most powerful reason is that, academic debate aside, other people believe the idea makes sense and has a reality for them. The academic challenge is to try to understand what that 'reality' might be for different people and to operationalize – to sketch the actual detail if you like – of that meaning.

People do identify with one another because of common locality or experience. In this simple way, people name that sharing by way of broad labelling or through 'signature' understandings such as 'my workplace', 'my hometown', 'my country' or 'my community'. Actual examination of the different meanings that people attach to these signature experiences may vary, and vary in contradictory ways, but that does not challenge their definition, even if its precision is problematic.

Wellman and Wortley (1990) have argued that friends and relatives are the principal means by which people secure support, but proximity plays an important role particularly outside kin relations. Locality still plays an important role here. But community may only be the key to signifying context of more instrumental sociological phenomena such as 'abundance' and 'strength of ties' (Wellman and Wortley 1990: 581). A more precise way of understanding how communities work may be in understanding 'networks' of relationships, and this term helps us overcome some of the problems of thinking about community 'boundaries' as fixed habitats and inward-looking relations. In fact people cross boundaries all the time, their identity as 'community' members blurs or changes from day-to-day depending on their changing locale and status within that community, and also on different issues which present themselves to them for daily or weekly consideration.

But whatever the academic debate about 'networks' or 'communities' most theorists agree that these terms and concepts present ways of understanding the *realities of daily support*. And participation and engagement provide, however these are produced, important ways that people create networks and support systems for each other. As Wellman and Wortley (1990: 583) argue:

> 'The networks are important to the routine operation of households, crucial to the management of crises, and sometimes instrumental in helping (people) change their situation. Many provide havens: a sense of belonging and being helped. Many provide bandages; routine emotional aid and small services that help (people) cope with the stresses and strains of their situations. A sizeable minority provide safety nets that lessen the effects of acute crises and chronic difficulties. Several provide social capital to change situations (houses, jobs, spouses) or to change the world (local school board politics, banning unsafe food additives, stopping cruelty to animals).'

In these above eloquent ways, communities ARE realities for most people outside academic circles, and so they make ideal sites for social changes which might improve health and end-of-life care.

The Compassionate City: a utopian project?

There is a long popular and academic tradition of employing the term 'utopian' as a pergorative dismissal of new ideas. However, utopian ideas were never meant, in the original meaning or in their political senses, to be unrealistic fantasies. Most utopian writing has a covert, sometimes overt, critical agenda. This means that much utopian writing has been designed as social criticism. By creating an ideal cultural or political set of stories or images, the authors or designers hope to show the inadequacies of the present while presenting other possibilities to their readers or listeners. Note that I employ the word *possibilities* here. Many a new idea began as a utopian one – especially social systems, from cities to democratic institutions to national socio-economic systems as diverse as capitalism and socialism.

In these ways, the primary function of utopian writing is not fantasy (which is frequently but not always its vehicle) but criticism and envisaging change. Healthy and Compassionate Cities are unashamedly in this tradition. Ashton et al (1986: 321), in commenting on the process of looking at fresh ways to look at health in the community at the Lisbon

Symposium in 1986, made the following pertinent remarks with respect to being 'realistic': They observe that there is a difficulty in:

'. . . reconciling the tension between imagination and realism which is the essence of planning. Although plans must be tempered by feasibility and resource availability, we must start by generating ideas – if we start with 'realism' we will never have vision.'

(From Ashton et al (1986))

The idea of the Healthy City and the Compassionate City falls neatly into a long tradition of attempting to envisage (to imagine) better, more humane and rational communities to live in (Eaton 2001). Cities such as Philadelphia in the USA or Canberra in Australia began their life as drawing-board utopias. Many architectural ideals and ideas were and are drawn from utopian images from the Aztecs or the European Renaissance, and although some have yet to see daylight many others have been unobtrusively integrated into contemporary plans and realities. Indeed, the majority of utopian societies are imagined as urban environments (Eaton 2001: 119).

Likewise much end-of-life care ideas also began life in utopian writings. Early echoes of palliative care can be found in More's *Utopia* and other ideas about voluntary euthanasia regularly arise in this literature from Anthony Trollope's *Fixed Period*, Ignatius Donnelly's *Caesar's Column* and again, even in More's *Utopia* (Carey 1999). Clearly, utopia does not equal 'unrealistic'. Utopian writing is critical writing, often by progressive thinkers, who prompt social and political changes through their writing. The Healthy City public health movement is part of this wider desire for constructive and practical change for the future.

Finally, Petersen and Lupton (1996) argue that, like much utopian writing, Healthy Cities are modernist dreams – they overrate the value of science, professional expertise and rational administration. I see no evidence that public health advocates of Healthy Cities overrate these attitudes, they merely aspire to them. The desire to see human action guided by a degree of epistemological certainty, as embodied in science and forms of reason, however imperfect, is to look and work toward a future time more free of self-interest and idiosyncratic decision-making than the one before.

Healthy Cities as marginal

If current Healthy Cities programmes are marginal, but the basic ideas are sound, we need to be working to make these programmes central and mainstream. If these ideas are indeed sound but interest is waning then this situation should be a prompt to redoubling our efforts to stimulate interest. Happily there is no waning interest in Healthy Cities, as more and more countries are adopting these programmes across Europe, Asia and the

Americas, and existing Healthy Cities are beginning new cooperative relations with other Healthy Cities (Baum 1998).

The abundance of interest is therefore a sound basis for addressing the marginality problem of some of these programmes. There has been recent discussion about how to tackle the problem of marginalization of Healthy City programmes in municipal government (Dooris 1999: 369–72). Dooris suggests that we need to overcome the view that Healthy Cities is a project rather than a central policy initiative for communities. We need to advocate the idea that Healthy Cities are an overarching, mainstream policy for councils and regional authorities.

Part of how to address this problem of mainstreaming is to develop strategies that will permit and encourage these authorities to increase their ownership of the programme rather than see it merely as a community participation project alone. We need to regenerate the debate about policy priorities in local government, particularly if we are to challenge the common view that economic development has a higher priority than health.

Finally, many authorities *have* put major work and commitment behind their Healthy Cities programmes, and have developed much valuable experience. Yet, there has been much less enthusiasm and interest from national and international quarters which could use and recognize that experience. As established Healthy Cities begin to reach out to each other and to those just beginning a programme, this will presumably become less of a problem.

The problem of evaluation

The problem of evidence is a fraught political and methodological problem, but much has been made of the methodological difficulties when these problems are clearly not the insurmountable ones. Baum (1998), for example, suggests a battery of methods and assessment points to evaluate Healthy City programmes. These methods include simple social surveys, epidemiological surveys, focus groups, key informant interviews, participant and non-participant observations, action research strategies, document analysis, and semiotic studies of media and other forms of popular culture. Baum favours a process approach to evaluation, using multiple methods to assess multiple processes and outcomes as a continual research act paralleling the life of a Healthy Cities programme.

Each of these methods is able to make distinct contributions to discreet aspects of the programme. Is social capital rising? Is knowledge about and access to services improving? Are major social groups as well as organizations participating in the programme? Are health policies being prioritized by authorities? Is health, by some measure or another improving or declining? Are people in general being supported in their loss? Do people in general *feel* that they are being supported in their loss?

The larger question of the *overall* effectiveness of a Healthy City programme can, to a large extent, be answered by recourse to the collective data about these kinds of discreet outcomes and issues. In these ways, we can give qualified and incremental answers to the greater question of the value of large, sociological approaches to public health. This reasoning has led some to already declare that health-promotion programmes such as those favoured by Healthy Cities are a success (Catford 1999). The fundamental methodological issue of evaluation is an issue confronting all good science, good medicine, good economic management and good city planning.

Behind this acknowledgement of the challenge and need for evaluation is the less acknowledged politics of knowledge. In each field just mentioned – medicine, science, economics and social planning – there is no suggestion that evaluation defines the limits to action. There is much of our scientific and medical work that is based on poor knowledge of effectiveness, a revised understanding about effectiveness, or a debatable, conflicting knowledge about effectiveness. Evaluation, in fact evidence, *informs* our actions because it cannot define them or we would have little to offer in science or medicine. Our strongest sources of certainty come from extremely well-controlled conditions where only a few variables are manipulated and examined, or they come from the hindsight of a history of trial and error.

This is the broader social and scientific canvas against which our best public health efforts must be read. In this context, we move forward with as much positive evidence as we can reasonably collect and agree upon, with as much positive desire to improve our collective lot as we dare express, and caution at all times as a vigilance against error and harm. Healthy City approaches are popular. They have some good evidence to support their practice but will require much more. In the meantime, we move towards our collective goals of community participation in health with reasonable caution and optimism.

Box 7 Criticism of Healthy City programmes

- The idea of community is a myth
- Healthy Cities are merely utopian visions
- Healthy Cities are marginal projects with waning interest
- How can we evaluate Healthy Cities?

In this chapter I have listed only the main features of Compassionate Cities, particularly their core concepts and characteristics. I have preferred here to show their theoretical ancestry, their conceptual tension within public health and palliative care, and to address the major criticism levelled at such ideas. In the next chapter I will elaborate on the social and policy meanings of the major characteristics of Compassionate Cities. I will take each characteristic and discuss what is meant by each of them with respect to the goals that each must set for the action strategies to be described in later chapters.

Chapter 4

Policies of Compassionate Cities

There is a fine line between visionary statements and practical policy. Broad policy visions of Healthy Cities are an important canvas that local communities employ to explore local problems and needs, and then develop the practical policy initiatives that address them. Nevertheless, the broader the policies the more susceptible these statements become to convenient accommodation ('we already do *all* this') and to radical appropriation ('we need to overturn our current practices').

Compassionate policies are based on Healthy Cities policies and the current social changes that most industrial societies seem to be undergoing (see Chapter 5). Such policies are meant as incremental, progressive reforms to our current public health vision that allow us to *build upon* current initiatives and to take this forward in matters to do with death and loss.

As with all public health initiatives and policies, we need to recognize at the outset that sound public health policy and planning more or less always covers matters to do with law and workplace policies, community education and awareness, and changes to media roles, activities and messages. In the pages that follow I will elaborate and expound on each one of the key nine Compassionate City vision policies by describing three or four operational policies. These operational policies supply a practical sense of direction for the vision policy to which they apply. Even if local communities have ideological or social difficulties or reservations toward any one operational policy they will still be able to discern, for their own practical purposes, the main spirit and direction of the vision policy to which these refer. These communities can then devise and initiate their own operational policies to implement the vision of compassionate public health underlined by that particular vision policy. I will now address each of the key vision policies and describe their accompanying operational imperatives.

Policy vision 1: Has local health policies that recognize compassion as an ethical imperative

Operational policy 1a: Fosters and supports educational initiatives linking health and compassion

There needs to be a public debate or some kind of community discussion forum about the value or need for compassion as an ethical imperative in the community. What is health? What is compassion? And what is one without the other? These are the crucial questions to ask about the nature of public health in the twenty-first century and their answers can provide a seamless basis for community policy and development that goes beyond the old welfare–health divide of twentieth century policy development.

This debate or community discussion forum needs to introduce and reflect about the absence of death and loss in current community policy and social development. As part of this period of community consultation, the pattern of death and dying and the morbidity of grief and loss can be introduced as ways of furthering, or even generating, the discussion about the practical role of compassion in their present community. This can also act as a basis for reflecting on current community needs in these particular areas of human experience.

An important element to any discussion about compassion and health, especially one that views death, loss and health in the context of continual changes in the life course (the constant cycle of beginnings and endings), is to highlight broader social questions: what kind of community do I wish to live in?; how do I wish people to behave toward me when death and loss confront me and those I love? From that perspective, and those questions, the need and the initial design suggestions for compassionate strategies can evolve.

Operational policy 1b: Fosters and supports compassion in the workplace, school and aged care facility

Each school, workplace or aged care facility must recognize that these are the great gathering places of people outside the home. Because of that sociological situation, specific strategies should be designed for each of them. Each site should be encouraged to have its own debate and discussion about the potential role of compassion in these habitats. And these sites need to establish an understanding of their own particular needs and possible strategies.

They may need to maintain a list of supportive services for their staff or pupils. These sites may also need to develop debriefing practices for sudden death or loss. They may need to establish peer networks of support –

'buddy' systems, mentoring programmes, or structured responses by staff and pupils towards other staff or pupils who experience loss or serious illness.

Whatever the practice choices or range of ideas that eventually become attractive to these habitats there needs to be a *written* workplace, school or aged care facility policy that can be revised and built upon by successive years or generations of pupils/workers. A policy is a living document that forms the basis of negotiation about shared needs. This cannot happen in any systematic or fair way unless this policy is available for everyone to see, and judge, for themselves.

Operational policy 1c: Fosters and supports health-promotion messages to incorporate death and loss

Most Healthy Cities, and many communities without this designation but who express and support health-promotion ideas and practices, need to incorporate the recognition of the universality of death and loss. This recognition should express itself in practical initiatives and educational programmes that facilitate community understanding of its own patterns of morbidity and mortality. A self-conscious community is a help-conscious community. An important part of this information is also the morbidity of grief and loss itself. Each community should attempt to understand the health consequences of death and loss on its members.

Furthermore, links should be made in education campaigns to permit people to connect their understanding about the impact of death with personal and social impacts of other 'endings'. The losses that people experience through death should be connected, if only symbolically, to other personal and community losses. Individuals and communities should not lose sight of the fact that forced separation from the things and people we love is at the core of our experiences of death and loss, and each commemoration of an important loss should remind us of the fragility of human life and its journey.

Finally, local governments must have community policies about death and loss. While it is common for local governments to have a disaster or civil emergencies policy (for bushfires, floods or terrorist attack) or public health policy (for infectious disease control), a policy about death and loss is much broader. Policies for death and loss recognize that we cannot control everything, and when deaths occur these experiences take a toll on a community's health and ability to work and play. A measure of a community's resilience and care is embodied in how comprehensive and active their policy development and partnerships around matters to do with the usual cycles of death and loss within their own communities are.

Policy vision 2: Meets the special needs of its aged, those living with life-threatening illness and those living with loss

Operational policy 2a: Fosters and supports the community awareness of the special needs of the aged, those living with life-threatening illness and those living with loss

Although we have made important inroads in promoting community awareness of the special needs of the aged, much more needs to be done around their social needs. We are yet to rethink issues around the institutionalization of the elderly and the importance and value of keeping these people in their own homes for as long as possible if that is their desire. In cases where medical conditions or disabilities prevent the maintenance of an accustomed lifestyle, integration into the local community will be essential if the social life of residents is not to deteriorate into a clinical-setting lifestyle of visiting hours, formal entertainment and visits from the local school children.

Residents in aged care facilities are not 'hospital patients' or 'impounded animals'. They are disabled or chronically ill members of a community that require special support but also *continuity of social relations*. The key challenge is maintaining existing relationships with friends, family and animal companions. Aged care facilities that do not cater for privacy, broad flexibility for visitors, the desire for meaningful work or animal companionship should be discouraged.

In addition to fostering and supporting the needs of the aged, there is also a great need to recognize and support the needs of those living with a life-threatening illness and those living with loss. The community awareness of the special needs of these groups of people is generally poor. The cycles of 'good' and 'bad' days for these people, what constitutes 'good' or 'bad' days, what things are helpful, and what acts and attitudes from others are not are important 'health-promotion' messages for the rest of us in assisting them. Our need for learning about these matters is generally great.

Operational policy 2b: Fosters and supports positive ageing, positive aspects of chronic illness and positive aspects of loss

In addition to identifying and understanding the diverse array of needs for this group, we also need to recognize that all these experiences are not uniformly negative. The community in general, and those affected, need to know this side of death and loss to bring balance to our understanding and our social responses.

Ageing is often associated with greater independence, not less. Dependency is about poor health not the simple facts of increasing age. Ageing, and also life-threatening illness, can bring greater values clarification for individuals – a clearer idea about what values, attitudes or even relationships are important, and which ones are not. Ageing is often associated with great experience in work or professional skills, in existential reflection and attitude, or in relationships. There is much that many sectors of the community can actually use from these generational assets in work, education and recreation.

In life-threatening illness, the overlooked is frequently re-examined. New if unwelcome experiences are accumulated by some that may be of use to others new to this experience, and whose fear can be addressed by those with more experience. New social and practical ideas to overcome disabilities can be invented by people who live with a life-threatening experience that few others may have thought of previously. The prospect of death can generate song, artwork, poetry or storytelling that benefits everyone. Many a new talent has been discovered in the shadow of death. These creative contributions are frequently prompted by a searching need or desire to express new thoughts and feelings prompted by this time.

And loss, like ageing and serious illness, can bring great sadness but also a renewed determination to honour legacies left in the wake of loss. In honour of memories of past tragic events, or dead friends and relatives, many people begin foundations, support charities or become advocates for reform that will prevent similar tragedies that caused the original losses. People living with loss can renegotiate the relationships with the dead, continuing that relationship in new ways, assigning these with new meanings. The dead can continue to be role models and significant others in death just as they might have done in life. These are positive contributions to self and community, and they derive from the under-recognized and positive dimensions of ageing, illness and loss (Kellehear 2002).

Operational policy 2c: Fosters and supports media recognition of their presence and experiences

It is important and valuable for people to see and hear their own experiences reflected back to them and to their loved ones. Such reflecting-back processes are personally reassuring and informative for everyone, but it also permits the whole community to understand its own fragility and vulnerability. This continual sense of fragility is important in maintaining a sense of compassionate purpose for any community, without which communities can feel that 'problems' are elsewhere 'out there' and not within. They are able to rally for their own and glean a more realistic and truly empathic understanding of mortal needs and trials by close contact and exposure to their own vulnerability. The media plays an essential role in that reminding and remembering process.

Communities must continually lobby, advocate and support initiatives in the local media (newsprint, TV and/or radio) for *regular* programmes that raise community awareness of the special needs and positives of ageing, serious illness and loss. Important to raising this community awareness and media willingness is the development of special 'days' or 'weeks' that celebrate, commemorate or highlight those needs. In this context, poster displays on billboards, festivals or use of celebrities at community functions all help promote compassionate ideas to the local media just as these do in conventional public health campaigns.

Policy vision 3: Has a strong commitment to social and cultural difference

Operational policy 3a: Fosters and supports anti-racist laws and inclusive policies; discourages religious discrimination based on class, gender, race and sexual preferences

There can be no safety, and therefore no genuine assurances, for public health if there is no community tolerance of difference. While we continue to see refugees or indigenous peoples as somehow less entitled to citizenship rights – as foreign or alien depending on the local language of exclusion – treatment of their health and illness, and their ageing and loss will be unfair. Inequalities are based on the belief that people are inherently unworthy, ineligible or even a direct threat to us because of class, gender, race, or sexual or religious preferences. This is an injustice unworthy of modern enlightened thinking.

In this context a compassionate public health is one that eschews any institutional or state-based policy that promotes inequalities and displays social and cultural intolerance. Religions that discriminate against women or other racial or cultural groups remain common. Religions that discriminate against gay and lesbian communities remain common. Workplaces that discriminate against certain classes or genders often do so in subtle ways which suggest cultural reproduction rather than overt discrimination. These practices can still be observed in many industrialized countries that have laws against these processes and acts. But they continue to happen. And as they continue to happen they continue to regenerate a regrettable level of loss and grief in the community directly related to the problem of exclusion. A compassionate policy can be developed in that shadow.

In this way, the progress of religions, schools and workplaces in general, in the matter of social and cultural difference, must parallel any progress in compassionate health policies. These matters are neither simple nor changeable by one or two community strategies.

Nevertheless, ALL strategies about death and loss must recognize and promote a discussion about the role of difference and social inclusion in effective public health programmes that aspire to address death and loss. Those verities always occur in a social and cultural context, and when these contexts operate in a national or local climate of inequality the existential problem becomes synonymous with the social and cultural one.

Operational policy 3b: Fosters and supports social and cultural differences in public education and school curriculum

The way that we respond to death and loss cannot be separated from the way we have come to learn about these matters. Our religions, migration or colonial history, or our placement in class or geographical position, will influence how we understand and what we understand about death and loss. In these ways, knowledge, like experience itself, is always 'situated'. In other words, our social positions influence our access to experience, information and knowledge generally. For some, death and loss is unfamiliar territory. For others, death and loss may shape the very character of their community, as indeed it does in some indigenous or gay communities.

We cannot be everywhere and cannot have all experience. School education is one of the few compulsory sites where we can learn about other people's experiences. Where the curriculum teaches about difference, the different experiences of death and loss may also be taught. In the normal course of public health education we may also learn from the death and loss experiences of most people in that community. Representation of that diversity in public posters and discussion, in media portrayal or in festivals and commemorative occasions is essential.

Operational policy 3c: Fosters and supports practices that recognize social and cultural influences in ageing, serious illness and loss in different groups

It is important for communities to learn that recognizing difference does not necessarily overcome stereotypes – it can also create them. Ethnic groups, gay and lesbian groups or age groups enjoy major diversity in values and attitudes. Migrant parents differ markedly from their children; their children differ in cultural persistence from their grandparents. As always, some things remain the same, others change. A gay man does not necessarily have the same identity, and therefore values and attitudes, of other men who have sex with men.

A compassionate approach to difference which develops practical approaches to that difference should embrace reflective practices that encourage people to assess their own assumptions and social presentation when interacting with others. It is important to learn about broad cultural matters of value and attitude when dealing with groups for which you have had little experience. But any public education campaign must also address *your own* differences so that you can better appreciate how your way 'creates' the impression of the differences in 'others'.

Operational policy 3d: Any implementation, policy or planning committee must include members chosen for their combination of skills, expertise AND social and cultural diversity

A key way that one can learn *from* others is to learn *with* them. With that principle in mind, any development committee should represent a diversity of people from the community that it seeks to support. Furthermore, some communities may be large and one might also consider developing separate compassionate policies within those communities. In other words, although there is definite merit in developing policies and practices that cut across whole localities in a municipal, it may also be effective and useful to develop culturally or socially appropriate policy or implementation sub-committees in particular communities within communities. The gay and lesbian networks may wish to identify their own needs around death and loss in a certain area and to feed their recommendations to the main municipal committee. Some ethnic or working class areas may feel the same.

Policy vision 4: Involves the grief and palliative care services in local government policy and planning

Operational policy 4a: Any implementation, policy or planning committee should include a member of the local hospice/palliative AND bereavement (sudden death) care team

This is recognition of the professional expertise and experience of those who have worked with people with life-threatening experience but also worked with those whose losses have occurred slowly over and beyond the course of their loved one's illness. A bereavement care worker may also be valuable to provide any policy or planning deliberation from the perspective and experience of one who has provided care for those whose loss was due to sudden death, e.g. suicide, accident or homicide.

The inclusion of these personnel allows any policy or planning to build upon the professional networks of these people, particularly in matters to do with health services and research information. Sometimes it may be possible to arrange to involve someone who has extensive experience with most types of death and bereavement. In this case a professional familiar with other kinds of death and loss (through family separation, dispossession or dementia) might instead be added to a committee for the additional and valuable experience they can contribute.

Operational policy 4b: Any implementation, policy or planning committee should include members with direct personal experience of ageing, living with a life-threatening illness or loss

This is recognition of the social expertise and experiences such a person may bring to this policy and planning work. The incorporation of personal experience may assist in building upon informal and/or non-clinical networks and partnerships. In a narrow sense this can be seen as 'consumer' representation, but more accurately, since most people bring their own experiences of death and loss to anything they do anyway, these persons serve to remind policy-makers in local government that such committees should be heavily community based in representation.

Operational policy 4c: Develops a local government policy to address loss and grief matters in the local community

As mentioned in operational policy 1c, it is imperative that local government develops a policy on death and loss in their local community. At all times this policy should begin with identifying community needs in an ongoing, participatory manner. Questionnaire surveys where the categories are researcher driven are poor community assessment tools. Participatory action research – a research exercise that is worked up with the assistance of the community itself – is the most desirable.

Once a broad range of needs have been identified, it is important that whatever service needs fall into the responsible areas of local government jurisdiction that these needs are addressed by that government. These service needs should be addressed as a normal funding matter for local government. Where no funding is available for any specialist services, appropriate application and lobbying in the usual manner should be attempted.

Any community development needs should also be addressed. In particular: the need for local education, information or awareness; the need for additional resources, personnel or financial; and the need for new partnerships and networks. All these service and community development needs, once identified by an initial assessment, should be part of the policy substance and rumination.

Finally, it is important that any developed policy recognizes the negative AND positive aspects of experiences in death and loss. No policy should assume, by innocent omission or professional ideology, that only negative experiences of death and loss should be subject to strategic policy development. People may need assistance in developing positive approaches or extracting the positive experiences from complex personal encounters with death and loss.

Policy vision 5: Offers its inhabitants access to a wide variety of supportive experiences, interactions and communication

Operational policy 5a: Fosters and supports media attempts to compare and contrast experiences of death and loss for its viewers and readers

There is a need for more public stories about ageing, living with life-threatening illness and living with loss, but more than this there is a pressing need for greater media *organization* of these stories. Currently, many countries actually do cover these matters but they occur at random, without warning, and are scattered anywhere in newsprint, TV and radio programming. While sport and world news commonly has its own section the problem of facing up to life in the shadow of death and loss does not. It is not true that these matters are always morbid, depressing or sad. Death and loss, like other parts of life, are often humorous, adventurous, inspiring, even amazing. Death and loss is news because it is not the same for everyone. Its contemplation has been a regular item in the New York Times Best Seller Lists over the years and the winner of the odd Pulitzer prize (e.g. Ernest Becker's *The Denial of Death*).

But some journalistic development of this material IS required for those interested in this compassionate policy. Cross-comparisons of experiences of living with a life-threatening illness and living with loss is needed. It is important to compare, for example, suicide with euthanasia (its act and its effects on survivors); living with cancer and motor neuron disease; bereavement with loss from dispossession or sexual abuse; the loss and grief of dementia (as sufferers and as carers); Red Nose Day with national Remembrance Days. Only by fostering these cross-comparisons do we best convert the compassion that death and loss generates in the community into a generalized set of attitudes and knowledge, which can emotionally and socially translate into supportive practices for the widest number of people in that community.

Operational policy 5b: Fosters and supports voluntary social services that assist people to maintain a preferred lifestyle in the face of death and loss

Volunteer services are key ways employed to rediscover community and reciprocity in modern life. We are familiar with volunteering for charity, e.g. for the sick and needy, but less so for each other. There is a great need and use for volunteer networks in loss and grief to provide support for people in similar situations. These networks can supply supports and comforts to and by people with shared experiences in common – parents of murdered children, families of suicides, or those suffering from dementia, etc.

The same observations can be made about volunteer supports for people living with life-threatening illness or in aged care. Hospice and palliative care services generally welcome volunteers but they are not always readily found. Aged care facilities frequently provide for 'community visitors', pet therapy programmes or programmes where ordinary neighbourhood dogs and cats are brought to visit the elderly who love animals. There are always needs for people who will read to those whose sight or reading ability has been compromised by disability or illness.

Volunteer services are worthy of support and fostering, for many people have no idea how they might contribute to the lives of people at the end of life, or are unqualified as professionals, or are unsure of how much they wish to help. Volunteer services are significant social avenues of health-promotion activity that supply the carers with support as they gently introduce themselves to community care. The support of these services is a crucial part of any Compassionate City policy.

Operational policy 5c: Fosters and supports special social support programmes for people in need

Volunteer services display a set of relationships where a willing and able person visits a willing person in some kind of need. Support – whether as a reader, a bringer of meals-on-wheels or a local animal companion – is brought TO someone. This operational policy suggests a reverse movement. People who live with life-threatening illness or loss and those who reside permanently in an aged care facility also have needs to contribute.

They may have a need to be actively involved in social occasions, to contribute to a workplace, to teach and learn, or to support others. In these ways, social support programmes may be workplaces, schools, churches or local government facilities that allow people who wish to contribute their services but who can only do so with active support from those institutions. Schools or workplaces, for example, can arrange transport to allow experienced and skilled frail-aged people to participate in workplace activities. These opportunities permit some elderly people to overcome the debilitating effects of institutionalization. Schools can invite people experiencing nursing home life, serious life-threatening illness or loss to speak to classes or teachers about their experiences.

On the other hand, these programmes may not exploit the experiences of age, illness or loss at all, but simply provide supportive experiences by way of voluntary work, teaching or participation to those for whom such experiences will be healing, comforting and/or morale enhancing. Supportive experiences are not simply experiences of providing services. They may also be experiences where we allow ourselves to be provided with services by those who have the same desire to be of use to others.

Policy vision 6: Promotes and celebrates reconciliation with indigenous peoples and the memory of other important community losses

Operational policy 6a: Fosters and supports national, state and local government initiatives and policies towards indigenous reconciliation

Many modern industrial societies have indigenous peoples who have experienced a long period of dispossession and maltreatment – Australia, Canada, North and South America, the Pacific nations, Japan, Africa and Malaysia to name just a few. Some of these countries have major reconciliation policies in place to heal the social and political wounds created by them. In Australia and the USA, for example, major federal policies and funding are deployed to address poor standards of living and health.

However, in Australia the Federal Government has consistently refused the indigenous peoples a national apology. Many small communities, especially rural ones, are critical of the social problems that they believe are created by their indigenous populations. This is also true of the USA. Yet the losses of these peoples are a matter of public record, as is their record of poor health, low life expectancy, poor employment and high crime rate.

The lack of local community recognition may be as important as a reticent national recognition of their losses. The academic research-based recognition of their losses is irrelevant beside their daily experience of alienation. Any Compassionate City that contains significant numbers of indigenous people must develop a local policy of reconciliation that is workable between all members of that community. Large steps are not required – some steps are.

Operational policy 6b: Fosters and supports an inclusive approach to Remembrance Days and festivals, including members from ALL sides of former conflicts, and former victims and workers of war

Once again, most countries have a national Remembrance Day that celebrates the memory of those who have died in past war and conflict. These days are about a national mourning over the loss of fallen comrades. They are also a day of celebration over matters to do with national autonomy, freedom and/or independence. In the past, these days have been days emphasizing victory or the birth of a nation, or men-of-war and their valour. In these ways, national days of remembrance are days of nationalism and social exclusion.

Compassionate City policies foster and support an inclusive approach to former conflicts and encourage organizers and participants to permit ALL sides to march and celebrate with them. These might also include recognition of the wartime costs paid by ALL people in a nation – men, women and children – as fighters, producers and family supporters. We might remember not only those who paid the 'ultimate price' for freedom but those who paid an expensive price as well – those disabled AND raped, those imprisoned, AND those who live with different kinds of loss brought by war.

ALL sides lose in a war and the part of Remembrance Day that honours loss should include all those that experienced those losses, and that includes former 'enemies'. Nationalism both heals and separates. Compassion, on the other hand, both heals and unites. A compassionate approach to Remembrance Days is essential in caring for all members of the local community by reminding them of their bonds with a world that grows smaller and closer every day.

Operational policy 6c: Has an annual day of remembrance for death and loss in peace times

Remembrance Days are one of the few national days where people are encouraged to think about death and loss. Unfortunately, that experience of death and loss is war related. In the twenty-first century we will need to move toward a more generalized Remembrance Day for all people. Because of the political significance of Remembrance Days it may be important to preserve this day for reasons of national unity and reconciliation. But another day of remembrance for death and loss in peace times is an important compassionate policy initiative. This can commence in any local community and can be commenced by creating partnerships with local organizations of bereavement care, hospice and palliative care, and major non-government bodies for the care and support of those with life-threatening illnesses.

On this day, all people who have experienced loss in peace times may participate in a public festival that recognizes the importance of their losses. These losses should memorialize all significant losses, including bereavement of human and animal relationships, losses of traditional lands and cultures, and other important symbolic endings that have created major trauma and sorrow for communities.

A compassionate approach to memorialization in times of peace should promote the idea that death and loss are universal experiences for all community members. As an important social and health policy, a national or local community day of remembrance helps us to share the sorrow and develop important, joint stories of healing. Only by this community sharing and recognition will we begin to see ourselves in the other.

Policy vision 7: Provides easy access to grief and palliative care services

Operational policy 7a: Promotes and supports a single telephone referral service for loss and palliative care

Compassionate local government policies should make access to grief and palliative care services in their area a priority. This should mean at least the promotion and support of a single phone number for these kinds of services. It may also mean web-page links from the main web page used for government services. However, a single phone number or web page does not automatically lead to greater access if the number or web page is not supported by wide advertisement of its existence. In this context, local workplaces, schools, churches or police stations and other emergency worker sites should display this information. The numbers and web sites might also be publicly displayed in signs at parks and gardens, or in street shopping centres or shop windows.

In the development of maximizing access to these services there needs to be some assessment about how relevant these services will be to the general community. Is the local hospice really only a cancer care service or is its remit wider? Is the local grief service really only a bereavement care service or is it wider? If these services are narrow services should they be supported to become wider in their community relevance? There also needs to be some assessment of community awareness: not simply of their existence but whether people know what these services actually provide for them? These social research matters go hand-in-hand with any policy development about access to these services.

Operational policy 7b: Promotes and supports local grief and palliative care services by facilitating access to schools and workplaces

Unless there is a serious attempt to mainstream grief and palliative care services, death and loss will always be viewed as abnormal social experiences in the community. It is essential that these kinds of services have ready access to schools and workplaces, both so that they can promote their services and provide support for these sites to inform themselves about death and loss. Partnerships can be created with these sites to develop social and personal capacity building – building personal and workplace abilities to deal with serious illness, death, or loss in the workplace or schoolyard.

Unless, we build a stronger and more participatory relationship with grief and palliative care services we increase rather than decrease our reliance on them, and minimize our ability to enhance our personal and community resilience and supports.

Operational policy 7c: Promotes and supports public education and awareness campaigns about the existence and nature of these services

Schools and workplaces are not the only areas of public life that require steady information about the availability and nature of grief and palliative care services. Many people do not work or attend schools and colleges. For reach to this wider group of community members broader community strategies are needed. Here, compassionate policies need to address the issue of promotion of these services. 'Sponsorship' of jazz, rock or classical concerts by services are good ways to advertise their existence and also to promote one-line understandings of those services. Because many of these services are not well funded it may need to be a local government policy to examine the possibility of subsidizing these 'sponsorships' on their behalf. Also, not every 'sponsorship' needs cash endorsements and sometimes festival, concert or show organizers will promote for community welfare in their own right.

Also important in these promotional contexts are the value of encouraging local service providers to be involved with local charities, schools functions such as fêtes, or community information or game nights, not for the purposes of fund-raising but rather for the purpose of consciousness-raising. Social functions can be arranged with other social clubs, and messages and ideas about death and loss can be integrated in informative, playful, even humorous, ways to the benefit of everyone involved. This promotion policy emphasizes new partnerships with social and business activities in the context of their leisure activities.

Operational policy 7d: Promotes and supports community initiatives from these services

Many services see their role in serious and non-reciprocal ways. These services are comfortable with 'talks' to the community, with fund-raising ventures for their hospice, or with promoting their service on radio. Few are actively engaged in programmes that might explore ways that communities might avoid using their services, or use them less than they might, or use them in strategic ways to enhance their own coping styles. How might a school deal with a sudden death *without* counselling? How might a neighbourhood keep an elderly neighbour in his or her own home for as long as he or she desires? What ways can people provide words of comfort to bereaved people without sounding banal or awkward or feeling anxious? What ways can people in workplaces or schools be *available* to those in grief or serious illness *without being intrusive*? What lessons have grief and palliative care services learnt that may be valuable to the wider community?

These questions highlight the need for clinical services to open up to a variety of social questions and philosophy of care that takes them away from a service orientation. Social care becomes a community capacity building exercise in the service of enhancing and strengthening people's own abilities and resources. Compassionate policies encourage access to grief and palliative care services in their own clinical terms but also in transformed public health terms. Clinical services are not enough. Social relevance is more than clinical services and a community development interest by these services will serve to encourage others to take a greater interest in their work. This interest can translate into use of those services in their own community terms and needs, rather than simply medical and other professionally defined ways.

Policy vision 8: Has a recognition and plan to accommodate those disadvantaged by the economy, including rural and remote populations, indigenous peoples and homeless

Operational policy 8a: Has a research-based understanding of the role of death and loss in the health and illness pattern of these communities

In any compassionate public health policy development there is a need for access to research-based information about death and loss in the nation, the state or province and, if available, the local area. It is important to understand how death and loss characterize particular group experiences in the community – the impact of AIDS, cancer or heart disease, or the medical, psychiatric or social impact of loss on sections of the community. We need to know about these kinds of 'global' knowledge but we also need to locally know about these experiences among our own people and localities. Sometimes this information will provide a sound foundation for policy direction but at other times it may not.

The gaps in our knowledge need addressing and so a part of any good policy development is also research development. A policy that targets a community-consciousness of its own experiences of death and loss needs to promote research into this area, if only to regularly ask and/or provide incentives of those who conduct research (services, colleges and universities or government departments) to examine or re-examine death and loss as a priority research area for the local area.

Operational policy 8b: Has a plan to address the death and loss issues for these communities

Marginal groups in the local community frequently have needs that require special attention and this may mean special policy attention to highlight the resource and personnel priorities for that area. Death and loss are not the same everywhere and its experiences in remote, rural or urban areas can have special difficulties, particularly if these are areas of considerable service deprivation. Often, geographically disadvantaged people live in communities where there is a high degree of resource sharing in services and in social networks, and specialized services can be difficult to find. A compassionate public health policy must examine these disadvantages and identify and plan around these problems (see operational policy 8c below).

Indigenous communities and the homeless also tend to be dealt with by specialized government departments or charities, and in these ways 'escape' mainstream attention from policy development and plans of action. This seems to be the fate of homeless populations in particular, although recently there have been hospice services for this population developing in North America and in Asia. Nevertheless, any policy development around death and loss must include a specific plan to address these matters in marginal populations.

Operational policy 8c: Promotes and supports grief and palliative care services for rural and remote areas, indigenous populations and the homeless

Aside from examining partnerships with other social and health services, and workplaces and church organizations, to explore ways to support marginal groups in the community to live with death and loss, a compassionate public health policy needs to ask several questions of its current local services. Do they have a service for the homeless? Do they have services for indigenous peoples? How culturally and socially appropriate are these services? What kinds of assistance, partnerships and supports are required for these services to perform their tasks adequately in these habitats? In what ways can local compassionate public health policies influence state, provincial or national policies for services in these areas and for these populations?

Operational policy 8d: Involves schools, police, churches, workplaces and businesses in the formulation and design of these understandings and plans

In any compassionate public health policy development, the use of palliative and grief professionals and some of those living with loss or life-threatening illness is essential. But it is also essential to include the larger part of the non-clinical service community in the development of these policies. The police and other emergency workers, businesses and churches are among the many sectors that need to be included in any policy and planning committee. Local policies must be 'owned' by a community, by which I mean that unless they feel these genuinely address local concerns in local and meaningful ways they will not be sustainable.

The use of key businesses, local service clubs and charities, universities and relevant government departments are also important to include because they are crucial resources for funding development. The implementation of policies will require financial and personnel resources and these must come from institutional contributions. The value of wide community inclusion for networking and resource matters is obvious. Senior and elite members of the community are important supports for any policy development with a desire for strong financial backing. Without a funding development plan, policies become mere wish lists.

Policy vision 9: Preserves and promotes a community's spiritual traditions and storytellers

Operational policy 9a: Fosters and supports inclusive religious politics, including ecumenicist and multifaith initiatives, but eschews the proselytization of tribal or medieval prescriptions

Some of the key storytellers in any community with a diverse and frequently helpful set of explanations, reflections and principles about death and loss are religions and spiritual traditions. Many Christian religions are embracing an ecumenicism (an attempt to explore common spiritual ground) and multifaith relations (a sharing and cooperation between very different kinds of religions), and design community celebrations and functions in this spirit. Where and when these festivals occur, from these outward-looking and cooperative religions, these should be supported. Where such movements and aspirations are present in a community's religions, the members of these congregations might also be encouraged to help plan or develop compassionate policies, which will enhance their ability to participate and support end-of-life care for all community members.

Senior members of these churches, mosques or temples may be invited to become members of any planning or policy committee, or alternatively perhaps a subcommittee devoted to making their own recommendations in their own right. However, religions that cannot participate in contributing to the wider community need without attempting to proselytize their beliefs to others, should not be enlisted for this work. Many people are insulted or made angry by attempts to convert them to religious beliefs, even though they may express interest in novel and useful ways of thinking and reflecting about suffering that a particular religion may offer. Restraint is essential in these matters today because all communities have many religions and followers and others do not subscribe to organized religions at all.

Operational policy 9b: Fosters and supports 'festivals of the spirit' in an inclusive context, which embraces religions and spiritual traditions both old and new

Many people are estranged from the mythological or spiritual traditions of their very own society because of early trauma or insensitive treatment in their early contact with organized religion, its instruction or its clerics. Others attend churches and temples but poorly understand the narrative (storytelling) basis of learning to make meaning from experiences of suffering.

An annual 'festival of the spirit' can alert people to the range of offerings within their own community, and provide them with an introduction to the rich tradition of ritual, theological, pastoral and social sources of comfort, meaning and thinking around the verities, including those of death and loss. Such combined festivals do much to promote multifaith cooperation and understanding, helping to allay and control community (and church) fears, prejudice or ignorance. These functions also help reconnect people to philosophies and stories that might actually be helpful to them if only they are able to rise above some of these long-standing early emotional and social reactions. Such regular activities are consistent and important to the promotion and support of the older traditions of storytelling and meaning-making, which is often less active and potent as a community aid as they might be.

Operational policy 9c: Fosters and supports the role of multifaith chaplaincy, pastoral care and humanist dialogue in their community role of comforting those living with life-threatening illness and loss

In colleges and universities pastoral care programmes are being developed, and where these are present it will be important that the local community has input to the curriculum development. Narrow curricula that are not ecumenical or multifaith in design will be less useful to broad communities characterized by multicultural populations. Where no such degree or diploma programmes exist, the development of compassionate public health policy may examine the feasibility of encouraging such training within the community, as a way of increasing the community development and social approaches to professional care that uses religious traditions as pedagogic basis of its learning and client supports. The local humanist, pagan or indigenous communities should also be encouraged and supported in publicly displaying and contributing their views to any curriculum development, community festivals or public discussions about the role of religion in community care.

Operational policy 9d: Fosters and supports the value and importance of spiritual beliefs and meanings in the development and support of healthy and compassionate lifestyles

The role of religion is important to health. Some religions support healthy lifestyles because of their support of particular dietary regimes. Others support emotional and social practices that are stress relieving and insightful, such as prayer and meditation. Still others promote new relationships with the dead and provide rituals that encourage a continuing bond with these former relationships. Others simply provide friendships and social supports at times when it can be difficult to find. In these simple ways, religions have much to offer each of us in times of crisis when we, or those we love, face death and loss.

No compassionate public health policy can afford to ignore the fruitful social and existential alliances that modern religions and spiritual traditions offer their communities. The Renaissance is over: for most industrialized nations Church and State are now separate. These are the times to forge relationships with formal religious systems on new terms. From them we may learn and attract new supports for our ideas and practices about compassion and health, ethics and personal meaning, social and spiritual supports. From public health and palliative care they may learn and find attractive new support for old ideas about equality, participatory politics, citizenship and tolerance of difference. Compassionate policies should make organized efforts to forge these new partnerships in any way that is mutually beneficial.

Old wine in new bottles: how new are these policies?

A superficial reading of the above suggestions may appear to many Western liberals as policies that reflect widely shared political and social ideas. However, a moment's thought will reveal them to be novel, even quite radical, in several policy and practice senses.

Firstly, both public health and palliative care do not currently share a policy space where end-of-life care is a joint concern. Palliative care finds health promotion a challenge in a context where they are more concerned about clinical services provision and development. And public health has been death-avoiding. The current compassionate public health policies do represent a new attempt to design policies that reflect potential concerns in a mutually relevant area – community care.

Secondly, although many, if not most, of these policies may be reflected in the state policies of some nations, many other nations will not share these views easily. The principles of power sharing, participatory politics, indigenous rights, multiculturalism, religious tolerance or tolerance of sexual diversity is news, even unpleasant news, for many countries and communities in the world.

Thirdly, of those nations whose intellectual, clinical and political elite share the values and specific policy aims of a compassionate public health, most of these policies, such as may exist in some form, will be federal/national or state/provincial policies. Their enactment and support at the local level may be quite poor, even absent. Local initiatives often reflect local interests, not necessarily state ones. And without local action and support, policies at any level are merely literary rather than social realities.

Fourthly, even in the most superficially tolerant societies there is much harmful – uncompassionate – conduct towards indigenous peoples and refugees, gay and lesbian communities and individuals, or the homeless. Churches are heavily derided, scorned or criticized; pagan or foreign religions unnecessarily feared or stigmatized; and sectarianism remains far too common. Death and loss remains widely excluded from everyday conversation let alone the workplace or schools. The negative aspects of these experiences remain overemphasized, leading to continuing high levels of fear, ignorance and dread.

Finally, compassionate approaches to community are not a recycled way of viewing 'community care', particularly if by that phrase we are referring to past social policy efforts to pass more of the responsibility for care on to 'families' – a strategy with serious implications for women. Williams (1989) has argued that the history of public welfare has been built upon the unpaid or low-paid work of women. This gender implication of past 'community care' policy development has been rightly criticized for its reductionism of 'community' to family, and from there to women. Compassionate Cities are social policies for everyone, i.e. men, women and children, at all sites – in workplaces, universities, churches and temples, shopping malls, sporting clubs and schools. Compassionate Cities are not community development initiatives that encourage end-of-life care responsibilities to return to women and families (Maclean and Groves 1991), although of course there is always a risk that some people may draw this kind of interpretation, so it is useful to disown, disavow and discourage this view at the outset.

The connection of death and loss to the wider problems of living together as communities in all our evolving, modern diversity is new. The linking of the idea of compassion to health, death and loss, and the reconnecting of death and loss to the broader experiences of change and endings, is news for many. All these linkages represent new ways to view and create community care at the end-of-life. These policies, and the novel connections they forge, do represent new challenges for communities, palliative care and public health. In the context of the history of the world, they also represent an old desire and ideal remade and rediscovered through the new gaze of a fledgling end-of-life care policy development.

Chapter 5

The social character of Compassionate Cities

What sociological foundations underpin a Compassionate City? Aside from its obvious theoretical links with public health ideas about Healthy Cities, how are the precepts for a Compassionate City actually derived? To put these questions another way, what is the contemporary 'real-world' basis for employing the language and ideas of Compassionate Cities? It is a simple matter to draw parallels between Healthy Cities and Compassionate Cities policies, but aside from internal theoretical consistency why are such policies needed in today's world?

For example, why should Healthy Cities that address death and loss be called 'compassionate' ones? Why does there need to be a commitment to social and cultural difference? For what reasons are our ideas about death and loss drawn to the plight of indigenous peoples, refugees or the unemployed and homeless? What is the point of preserving and promoting spiritual traditions and storytellers in the context of an increasingly secular society?

In this chapter I will identify some answers to these questions. In order to do this I will begin this chapter by highlighting some of the key observations by current social theorists about life in today's industrial societies. I will review the theoretical meaning of some of the key descriptors of modern society as employed by these theorists – risk society, network society, the Third Way, and globalization – and show how these concerns underpin the idea of the Compassionate City. I will also critically identify where current social theory and comment fails to anticipate and explore ideas about Compassionate Cities that are relevant to its own definitions of our current problems and solutions.

Finally, I should preface this chapter with one qualification. Contemporary social theory and debate is interdisciplinary and complex. I do not mean to summarize the comprehensive intricacies of this debate or theorizing. My purpose is to merely provide a simple indication of the kinds of concerns that now occupy and exercise the current generation of social theorists. I do this to provide readers who are not familiar with these social debates with a sense of the cultural legitimacy of current public health ideas, including those that address issues of death and loss such as the current Compassionate Cities approach addressed here.

Of current troubles

Most social theorists agree that we now live in a 'postmodern' or 'postindustrial' society, a society characterized by 'reflexive modernity' and 'globalization'. The collapse of Soviet communism seems to have settled the debate about which economic system will lead us through the twenty-first century – state-controlled economics is out, the free market in all its variations and glory seems to have won the day. Not so, however, the social and political debate about the 'good society'. How we should live, and what civil, political and moral conditions still occupy the thoughts and books of all leading social theorists of the day (for an excellent review of this literature see Turner and Rojek 2001)? Although there is debate about the specifics of a diagnosis of our current moral and social conditions, and widely different views of what is to be done, there is a broad consensus about some of the basic features of our current troubles.

We live in times of industrial modernity but the period of 'industrial' modernity has had two phases, an 'early' and a 'late' modernity. In early modernity, from the Industrial Revolution until the turn of the twentieth century, people sold their labour to industries that, in their turn, paid workers from a portion of their profits. Industry sold and priced their products in the marketplace on the basis of scarcity. In other words, the measure of a product's value was based upon their naturally occurring marketplace scarcity (e.g. gold or oil) or their socially constructed scarcity (e.g. land, professional services or citizenship). The struggle between capital (those who owned the means of production) and labour (those who literally became these means) was a struggle over the terms and conditions, or the risks and benefits, and how these were to be distributed. Questions about how the risks and benefits are distributed, and to whom, are central to the moral problem of social power and inequality. In early modernity, these problems were formulated by many social observers (e.g. Marx, Weber, Veblen, etc.) in collectivist, social-class terms based on common, shared experiences of ownership or the workplace.

The accumulation of wealth during the twentieth century rose sharply. Economic development paralleled scientific and technological development, each enhancing the other in a spiral of complementary investment. As the technical and economic development increased so too did the needs and skills of workers within those key industries who were able to produce and maintain them. The factory worker soon became the clerk and the clerk soon became the professional. This occurred in the space of a few generations. In the late twentieth century – sometimes referred to as late modernity – we arrived at the point that Beck (1992) calls 'reflexive modernity'.

'Reflexive modernity' emerged as a phrase to describe what happens when people are continually prompted to become aware of the personal and social conditions of their life course. Furthermore, this type of self-consciousness comes about because the predictable stages, social values and rituals (social norms) of the life course break down. This break down creates a widespread need for people to individualize, or to put it another way, to personally tailor and steer their lifestyle in a broader cultural context of disorder and uncertainty. This society-wide disorder and uncertainty are created, and continue to be created, by the following conditions.

Firstly, rising education levels cause people to think about the state of the world and their place and identity within it – in other words, to be reflexive. That is, rising levels of information and inquiry about things in the world encourage one to self-monitor and self-analyse. The scientific/rational mindset is now no longer simply an applied part of scientific occupational territories such as physics or chemistry, but also medicine, social and behavioural sciences, management and commerce, engineering and information sciences. The so-called 'information society' means that *knowledge* and *analysis* are not merely occupational or elitist qualities produced by academics, scientists and professional classes. They are also endemic social attitudes and cultural values. They are shared assumptions and storylines about everyday life for most people. Science, industry or medicine no longer have a monopoly on rationality. These are domestic and private qualities of the modern individual.

Secondly, whilst in early modernity a person had, or expected to have, one career, one marriage and one religion, today people have, or at least consider the possibility of having, multiple careers, marriages and beliefs. Identity is not necessarily tied to work, family or nation in any singular, linear understanding of those spheres of social experience. The diversification of the workplace and work practices increases the likelihood that class experiences will not necessarily be based on shared experiences of work.

International migration, secularization and globalization of capital have also created a diversification of ideas about work, family and nation. The idea of progress – in one's personal life, in one's career or in the life of a nation – is now precarious, changeable, diverse and conditional. Having a steady job and spouse no more predicts a safe and stable future personal life any more than a strong science and industry predicts a secure national one. The international movement of human beings, finance, education, entertainment products, terrorism and social protest permeate and transcend national borders.

Thirdly, contemporary health, sexuality, social movements and politics create complex and multiple aspects of identity and not merely fixed states. 'Who am I?' is an ongoing question and a major personal and marketing problem. Identity is contingent (upon contexts rather than a particular inherited status), fragile (subject to change) and vulnerable (to psychological and social damage). Although the old statuses of feudal and early industrial societies (e.g. gender, class and race) still exert an influence on one's identity and life chances (e.g. access to scarce resources such as wealth or services), a reflexive modernity thrusts new ideas about risk and benefit that cut across these categories. Class or status does not solely determine 'risk' any more. Risk – the probable harm from technological or social processes – can affect anyone. Pollution, chemical damage of foods, acts of terrorism, even sexually transmissible diseases, can affect anyone in spite of their class, sexual orientation, wealth or geographic location.

Finally, Castells (1996, 1997, 1998) has argued that late modernity is witness to a new 'social formation', a new global social system. It makes no sense to think of ourselves purely in terms of the old industrial social divisions any more. We are witnessing the rise of 'informational capitalism'. This is a time when workers trade in knowledge and information across a wide range of social and economic networks. There is an increasing personal investment on consumption and lifestyle rather than work. People now take a more instrumental view of work – they work to gain an income that will support their emotional investment in a particular personal lifestyle that may bear no direct relationship with work itself. Their sense of solidarity – their sense of community and identity – frequently lie with the deeper friendships and relationships of their private lives rather than, as they previously did, in their work lives.

The problem of power is also no longer simply hierarchical. Information sharing, strategic positions within an information circuit and network alliances outside workplaces or globally within them, can both strengthen and destabilize local power relations. People are able to work *across* the up and down traffic of the exertion of authority to undermine or support formal decisions and practices. The Internet, social movements, individual worker contracts, work-related migration, international networking, and media and popular culture are all sources of alternative power to traditional forms of authority and capital. Whereas formerly a worker with a grievance had only their trade union to represent them, today several equally potent political options present themselves through litigation through the justice system, media representation and coercion, and political lobbying.

But this reflexivity – this self-awareness and individual charting of life courses – also highlights the problem of risk in the modern world. Although great freedoms may come to those who successfully steer their own course through work and family life, there are also great social, psychological and physical risks and costs. Beck (1992) has argued that many of the key social institutions that were created to manage risks are paradoxically themselves chiefly responsible for their creation. Science and medicine, public health and industry have all been implicated in both identifying and creating risk.

Unfortunately, governments and industry have been keen to assert authority over the determinants of risk, arguing that they or their 'experts' are able to arbitrate and measure potential harm to individuals and communities in matters to do with their products. The knowledge of 'families', 'patients', 'students', 'workers', 'residents' or 'consumers' is considered less authoritative in matters to do with the environment, health, research or industrial development.

The sociological problem with this dismissal in the context of reflexive modernity is that these shallow social categories disguise multiple identities within them, literally hiding a labyrinth of great social, cultural and professional diversity. The poor or non-responsive approach of government and industries to these audiences have led to major growth and influence of social movements and alternative lifestyles, and a deepening of political engagement and civil disobedience. Underlying and cross-cutting these historical and political scenarios, according to Turner and Rojek (2001), lie even more fundamental, cross-cultural tensions between all human communities.

First, there is a tension between scarcity and solidarity. Scarcity is the watchword for the economic observation that there are limited resources in the world. This creates competition for their gain. For some social theorists, this has led to an evolutionary theory of 'survival of the fittest'. Turner and Rojek (2001) argue, however, that being fit is always temporary because we all age and die, and these facts in those close to us stimulate sympathy as well. Such obvious social experiences such as shared experiences and sympathy can lead to cooperation, resistance, trust, innovation and change – or to employ another word, solidarity.

The tension between scarcity and solidarity is experienced by the individual as 'reflexive embodiment'. This means that men and women experience the world through their body: through its physicality, and also through its social and political presentation to others, namely gender, race, disability, age, etc. This idea of 'embodiment' is the idea of the body-in-the-life-course; a vessel subject to change, and changing social and political categorization by oneself and others.

This contingent quality of embodiment – the way our bodies feel to us and appear to others – contributes to reflexivity, the modern psychological condition of self-monitoring and self-analysis. It also leads to a sense of vulnerability, an acute awareness that social events and processes may damage us. Seale (1998), like Becker (1973) some 30 years before him, argues that this vulnerable condition of embodiment, the organic susceptibility to death, is the main driving force behind all social and cultural activity. This awareness of vulnerability has ensured that despite the rising popularity and engagement with a rational/scientific discourse, most people also use and support irrational/religious knowledge as guides to their private decision-making and attitudes.

From these above observations of recent history, political economy and sociology we can identify five central problems of reflexive modernity that any programme of social reform needs to address. These are: (1) the need to revise our understandings of inequality to include the casualties of globalization, e.g. Third World, indigenous peoples, or homeless; (2) the need to revise our understanding of community from a system that is closed and exclusive to one that is open and inclusive; (3) the need to incorporate the fact that despite the rise of the rational/scientific imagination, the popularity and attachment to the irrational/religious imagination remains strong and sustaining to most populations; (4) the need to revise our understanding of power relations from one that is hierarchical to one that takes account of the power of networks; (5) the need to incorporate the idea of contexts to any programme of change and innovation – the influential role of settings or environments – whether these be to workplaces, homes, human bodies, forests or the oceans, all are important to human safety and well-being. I want now to show how a leading critic and social theorist has developed his major theory of future social reform by addressing these same five problem issues of reflexive modernity.

Of solutions

Recent sociological and political recognition of these developments and problems has obviously led to revised ideas about social democracy and political participation. Political solutions to address issues of power and inequality, national identity and security, public health, community policing and surveillance, and ethical matters about science and industry have undergone major rethinking.

Writers such as Beck (1992) and Giddens (1991, 1998, 2000) believe that political terms such as the Right and Left no longer represent substantive political categories. These are now empty categories. Modern public health, environmental issues, sexual and ethnic identities, international migration and refugee movements, the international spread of capital and social values and attitudes (globalization), all point to political analyses – and reform agendas – that must transcend the old industrial understandings of labour (the obsession of the Left) and capital (the obsession of the Right). Of particular relevance is the way in which the global movement of investment capital has created dispossession among ethnic minorities and indigenous peoples around the world.

Castells (1996) speaks of the network society in this connection: a society of linkages put together for specific purposes and that dissolves when the project or purpose for that network is complete. His three-volume analysis of the politics of information – tracing exactly how knowledge itself is power – and the globalization of industry and identity in the information age is a descriptive tour de force. But Castells' magisterial analysis (Castells 1998: 389) of the way things are self-confesses no solutions. Giddens (1998, 2000), on the other hand, speaks about the Third Way – a 'centre left' brand of politics that has often been accused of the left moving right! What is the 'Third Way' and how does it attempt to address the needs and structural problems of reflexive modernity?

Third-Way politics is a political position designed to move beyond the old-style socialist left. It is a position that refuses inequality but accepts market economics. Its valuable continuities include a concern for equality and protection of the vulnerable, and freedom as autonomy. Third-Way policies advocate no rights without responsibilities and no authority without democracy. Finally, societies should be philosophically conservative, adopting a precautionary view of the ambiguous consequences of development. They will also exhibit cosmopolitan pluralism, a multiculturalist idea of citizenship exhibiting multiple ethnic and national affiliations (Giddens 1998: 66).

Central to Third-Way policies is the need to renew civil society, particularly through partnerships with government; community renewal through local initiatives; an involvement of the voluntary sector; and protection of the local public sphere (Giddens 1998: 79). Such policies call for recognition of the centrality of ecology and environment; the spread of political engagement; the need for participatory politics; institutional individualism – a recognition that most rights and entitlements are designed for individuals rather than families, and these presuppose employment, education and mobility (Giddens 1998: 36); and multicultural nationalism and citizenship, what Giddens refers to as 'cosmopolitan pluralism'.

We can see that each of these calls for recognition acknowledges the problem of reflexive modernity. The centrality of ecology and environment acknowledges the central role that settings play, as supports and as casualties, in technological innovation and industrial development. The recognition of the spread of political engagement, and of the need for participatory politics, is recognition of the influence of networks and the need to revise our ideas about inequality and community as problems of social inclusion.

The call for recognition of institutional individualism and multicultural ideas of citizenship affirms the need to make communities work as open and inclusive networks rather than closed and exclusive ones. But this recognition also underlines the point that old ties and allegiances to collectives such as class or ethnic groups are now overlaid by a diverse and competing group of identities. Either/or categories must be both/and groupings if new and sustainable groupings are to have any chance of survival and coherence.

Of continuities

Employing these same criteria of relevance to today's problems of reflexive modernity, how do the theoretical features of Compassionate Cities address these sociological problems and to what extent, if at all, do these features complement the solutions touted?

If Turner and Rojek (2001) are right in their view that the experience of vulnerability is a cross-cultural problem for all communities, they are also right in observing that competition is not the sole way communities cope with scarcity. The precariousness of everyday life is indeed managed by other social strategies, including empathy, cooperation, reciprocity and other forms of social sharing. In this theoretical context, 'compassion' may be said to be the public health umbrella concept for these collective terms that sociologists call 'solidarity'.

If we are to accept that market economies are to rule our lives, then the political and social challenge is to address the problems inherent in these systems as systems that create inequalities. The concern for these inequalities and their health consequences has been a long-standing concern of all public health initiatives, and is recognition that inequalities create an uneven distribution of risks and hazards for the poor and marginalized within a country but also in global terms. It is also recognition that access to help – to health and human services and products that will address those problems – are also compromised by economic market forces. This is the wider context of the politics of public health and points clearly to the need to recognize contexts (settings and environments) as the crucial units of analysis in determining the health of any peoples.

This principle applies without qualification to death and loss. In this case, a Compassionate Cities approach to death and loss only makes sense if identification of needs and problems (and solutions and actions) are based on the assumption that compassion is not simply a human sentiment but a holistic/ecological idea tied to social settings and systems. If compassion is an ethical imperative for health it is so because the need for empathy, cooperation and reciprocity must extend beyond health to include the most tragic and poignant experiences beyond it, death and loss. These are undoubtedly the human needs that emerge in the darkest hours of human suffering. In these ways, Compassionate Cities must have *local health policies that recognize compassion as an ethical imperative.*

There are other continuities in our current troubles and solutions, as identified by recent social theory. The idea of compassion as solidarity, as a basis for identifying with those whose ability to compete in the market system is compromised, is to create a recognition beyond the conventional social divisions often identified by social theorists. Most critical social science employs the plight of women, particular ethnic groups, or poorer social classes or countries as their chief examples of marginality. Occasionally the mentally or physically disabled are identified for the purposes of this argument or illustration. It is uncommon for mainstream social theory in particular to devote itself to a consideration of mortality. Turner and Rojek (2001), for example, write about vulnerability in terms of the human understanding and sympathy of disabled and ageing people. Death, on the other hand, barely rates a mention beyond the banal observation that '. . . human beings are subject to death' (Turner and Rojek 2001: 123).

But those ageing, others who live with a life-threatening illness and those living with loss are also people with special needs that are currently provided little support beyond direct services for the most troubled among them. Although aged care has become an increasingly important area for policy development, and the 'grey' vote of industrial societies has ensured a steadily increasing political recognition, the same cannot be said about the other two social categories. There is little recognition that people living with loss and those living with life-threatening illness have needs beyond simple medical ones. Bereavement, for example, is considered to have acute problems requiring health services intervention for some of the more 'complicated' or 'abnormal' responses. The social needs of the bereaved are rarely considered in the medical literature and they are absent in public health discourse.

The problem of inequality around matters to do with health and those ageing, living with a life-threatening illness and loss are crucial in expanding our understanding of social justice and those social categories. However, this does not mean that other more conventionally recognized populations are any less important. In this context, Compassionate Cities *recognize and plan to accommodate those disadvantaged by the economy, and these include rural and remote populations, indigenous peoples, the unemployed and the homeless.*

Notwithstanding this commitment to these above populations, Compassionate Cities must *meet the special needs of its aged, those living with life-threatening illness and those living with loss*, because in these times of reflexive modernity we need to revise our understanding of inequalities. An inclusive strategy to address inequalities, such as the Third Way or public health approaches that address modern social analysis, is a strategy that recognizes that power creates casualties *across* as well as below the hierarchical structures of a social and political system. People can feel disenfranchised, can have fatal consequences following bereavement, and can experience abandonment and rejection from cancer or AIDS just as surely as unemployment, homelessness and other forms of dispossession that can also create these experiences.

Compassionate Cities must also *have a strong commitment to social and cultural difference* because the basis of modern citizenship is based on a growing recognition that we are moving towards societies whose citizens have multiple identities. And also we need, because of this growing multiculturalism and the fact that work and community are based on social networks, to create reform programmes that recognize the need to make communities ones that are inclusive and open rather than exclusive and closed. In this context, Compassionate Cities are cities that rely on, indeed assume, that communities are network based, open, and inclusive of social and cultural diversity.

Compassionate Cities also *offer their inhabitants access to a wide variety of supportive experiences, interactions and communications.* This is crucial in a time where the populations themselves are extremely diverse and cosmopolitan. On the one hand, the normalization of death and loss require strategies that mainstream these experiences in the popular media (in theatre, newsprint, radio and television). However, the Internet, workplace and other major recreational venues where people place their greatest emotional investments – family, friends, church and sporting circles – are also crucial as supportive places. These sites are well understood modern health-promotion sites but they are yet to become places where learning and support about death, dying and loss can take place in a manner that treats these matters as *life* matters rather than as morbid, 'last-thing' matters.

Finally, there is one final characteristic of Compassionate Cities that addresses the problems of reflexive modernity and act as theoretical continuities for any reform agenda that aspires to social justice. Both the cosmopolitanism and scientific/rational agenda of late modernity point to a simultaneous tension between a loosening and strengthening of traditional ties.

On the one hand, industrial populations are growing accustomed to working and playing in contexts of great social and cultural diversity. The growth of interest and state commitment to human rights and citizenship is at least partly about creating political ways to address problems of inequality that transcend matters to do with the old industrial social divisions such as wealth, race or gender. As Giddens (1998: 105) puts it, any revised understanding to the former notion of equality as sameness must include the notion that a concern for equality must begin with a commitment to *inclusion.* In this context, communities are networks joined together by local and international networks, which preserve identity at the same time as that identity becomes blurred with other traditions. These diverse cultural influences may emerge from a new adopted society, foreign media incursions (and values) in one's birth society or the cultural persistence present in parental and family relations. Whatever the sources of dissonance and resonance, reflexive modernity now creates a cultural scenario where there can be few certainties about the source of any particular social locality's moral and cosmological inspiration.

On the other hand, even among those whose entire biography and family traditions have been within a Western, industrial tradition, significant commitment to religious traditions exists and proliferates. The so-called scientific/rationalist imagination is not a *replacement* imagination but merely an additional mindset. The religious imagination is alive and well, with most people committed to different types of religious belief.

Furthermore, there has been a major revival of commitment to 'New Age' beliefs – an amalgam of Eastern religions, paganism and spiritualism. Such mixtures of new and old religions act as an adjunct to the scientific imagination by supplying moral or ethical guidelines. These sometimes coexist with political beliefs about how the world should be, although sometimes they may occur without these supplements. The Compassionate City characteristic that *preserves and promotes a community's spiritual traditions and storytellers* recognizes this cultural tension and paradox within the context of reflexive modernity.

In the above ways, we can see the obvious continuities of the characteristics of Compassionate Cities with the spirit and rationality that currently underlies our understanding of reflexive modernity. Nevertheless, there are important elements missing within the current round of prominent social analysis. Not all characteristics of Compassionate Cities represent continuities with our current understanding of our problems and solutions, notwithstanding the very general level at which these are identified. There are three major omissions in current contemporary social analysis and theory that do not anticipate the reform agenda of Compassionate Cities. These omissions include the centrality of death and loss in human experience, the link between death-related loss and other kinds of loss, and the rising global importance of hospice and palliative care services.

Some missing elements

Contemporary social theorists neglect the subject of death. I am not referring to those who work in specialized areas such as the sociology of death but to mainstream social theory. If 'death-denial' as a phrase ever had any legitimate social cache it applies in this area of human activity. Social theorists write about human activity as if they and their human subjects never die. When one of their kind condescends to write a special book on the subject of death and dying (e.g. Elias 1985) it is, curiously, to merely speculate about the experiences without recourse to previous academic work on the subject.

Among Anglo-European social theorists only Bauman (1992) has protested at this neglect of death in social theory. Notwithstanding the accuracy of his observations about the silence surrounding death in social theory, he also ironically ignores the empirical social science research into death and dying that he berates his theory peers for ignoring. Like Becker (1973) before him, Bauman (1992) sought to '. . . blow the whistle on the marginalization of death within disciplines like sociology' (Beliharz 2000: 146), but unfortunately this didn't extend to actually looking at the death scholarship his other colleagues were producing outside of social theory itself.

General work about the problems of modernity and its futures tend not to mention death. When they do mention death these writers frequently keep its nature vague, with mortality figures or allusions such as violence, disease or 'risk'. At other times the idea of death is employed as a background idea, such as Giddens' (1991) concept of 'fateful moments' – occasional social experiences of crisis that bring one's life into sharp relief. In a later work, Gidden in his book *The Third Way* (1998: 121) referred to death in just this style:

> 'Burke famously observed that, "society is a partnership not only between those who are living, but those who are living, those who are dead, and those who are to be born". Such a partnership is presumed, in a relatively mundane context, by the very idea of collective pensions, which act as a conduit between generations. But an intergenerational contract plainly needs to be deeper than this.'

Two observations can be made about Gidden's 'brush' with the subject of death in this above quote. First, his example of pensions, however, mundane, is an example of abstractifying death – death is a generational phenomenon. In this analytical context, it is an historical rather than personal attribute of social life. Second, the example of pensions as an example of a social partnership between the living and the dead is truly a 'mundane' context. The idea that death and dying may leave social legacies in the minds and social actions of individuals and generations that transcend the banalities of pensions is never realized or described in even the most basic ways.

How the personal and social experience of loss acts as an impetus to a diverse range of social movements in times of war and peace is not described. The way that the meaning of death creates further experiences of death, loss and protest among indigenous peoples is not described. The way that the human experience of death and loss generates greater social, financial and personnel support, and production for popular, scientific and medical cultures. How fear of death, even how death heightens a community's sense of vulnerability (erodes or strengthens its sense of solidarity), these roles for death and loss are not articulated or connected to other social forces.

Castells spends three volumes outlining the forces that drive and characterize the information age, but nowhere does he speak of the role or impact of two world wars, the holocaust or the threat of nuclear extinction on recent technological or industrial initiatives, or social movements. The fear, rather than mere incidence or prevalence of AIDS or cancer, seems to play no role in the political and social motivation of nation states, their industries or sciences, in the development of infrastructures, policies or product lines in medicine, education, welfare or industry. Despite discussions about AIDS, infant mortality, massacres or killings (these are indexed terms) the *experience of death and loss* as personally real and socially fertile facts of our modern existence do not figure in his analysis. And yet, paradoxically, the final lines of his acknowledgements thank his surgeons for giving him '. . . the time and energy to finish (his) book' (Castells 1998: xiv).

'Risk society' has no meaning if the final destination of risk itself is not recognized to be death. Reflexivity is too shallow, lacks political and onto-logical depth, if its self-analysis and monitoring do not include the facts of death for self and those we love. No theory of vulnerability makes sense without recognition that this fragility points to the collective and personal possibilities of extinction. Whether we speak of social theorists or the very idea of citizenship, any denial of our ultimate destinies as fragile, interde-pendent organisms is a dangerous political and analytical omission. The facts of social solidarity – the sociological meaning of compassion – *implies a concern for the universality of death and loss*, and this is central to Compassionate Cities.

Crucial to our emergent understandings about death and loss is the par-allel recognition of the symbolic and physical continuities of death and loss that go beyond biological death and immediate experiences of bereavement. Death is about irretrievable, irreversible endings. Biological death is an obvious example and its effects on survivors in the bereavement experience are all too obvious. Less obvious, but equally consequential, are other kinds of death. Dispossession and cultural destruction is one of these. Examples include the dispossession of indigenous populations and the collective mem-ory of death and betrayal. This legacy of death and broken trust must be factored into any analysis of lower life expectancies and morbidity burdens. Both physical and psychiatric consequences of dispossession in these popu-lations, but also those of refugees, free migrants and abused populations such as victims of torture or sexual abuse, must be linked to the morbidity and mortality of loss.

The losses of one's country, ancestry, traditions or core self-identity are deaths and losses that must be connected to our traditional ideas about bio-logical death. The future and quality of end-of-life care must incorporate recognition that end-of-life experiences are inclusive experiences of death and loss experienced more broadly. A literalist position about death and loss as biological death and immediate bereavement may be appropriate for palliative care but not for a public health end-of-life care that is inclusive of compassionate ideas and actions within the community. *Compassion is a holistic/ecological idea* and *promotes and celebrates reconciliation with indigenous peoples and the memory of other important community losses.*

Finally, hospice and palliative care services are growing in international importance. At the same time, public health and health promotion grows in global importance. While palliative care becomes more attracted, almost daily, to the idea of the immediacy of dying, death and loss, public health continues to see its service to the world in terms of the prevention of illness or quality of life enhancement of those with chronic illness. On the one hand, we have a service developing around terminal illness rather than life-threatening diseases, and bereavement care after cancer deaths rather than grief and loss care as a result of any kind of death. On the other hand, we have a public health approach that does not, as yet, recognize experiences of dying, death and loss as matters of direct public health policy and action.

Similar to the funeral industry, grief and palliative care services are commonly viewed as important but socially awkward. Death creates uncomfortable social reactions and ambivalence, and the services designed to deal with them are not untouched by these tensions and stresses. The services occupy a similar moral and cultural position to women's refuges or shelters for the homeless. The staff who work in these places are heroic, selfless and dedicated but they are widely seen to be places not to be visited by the faint-hearted. The services exist to some extent on the failure of our normal social arrangements to develop appropriate structures of care in the normal and usual contexts of a citizen and their networks – a social observation well described by advocates of normalization theory.

Notwithstanding the current cultural position of much current grief and palliative care described above, we must also recognize that these observations do not exhaust the therapeutic approaches taken by these services. Outside of hospice and acute care settings, for example, many palliative care services strive to incorporate themselves into the usual routines and social networks of the people for whom they care. To the extent that they are able to do this, to the extent that they are given the resources to try and to the extent that they are able to articulate the care philosophy, these services have a wealth of de facto 'public health' experience in care of the dying.

Outside of conventional counselling scenarios, beyond those whose needs are well served by professional responses to grief care, many other grief workers work with communities to support those living with loss. To the extent that they are able to do this, to the extent that they are given the resources to try and to the extent that they are able to articulate the therapeutic value of community and peer work in loss and grief, these are de facto 'public health' experiences of care with those living with loss (Groopman 2004). In these particular community ways, the support, recognition and *easy access to grief and palliative care services* are crucial to any Compassionate City approach.

Towards a compassionate society

Identifying the contemporary social character of Compassionate Cities suggests a number of broader observations about their policy features.

Compassionate Cities in the context of the 'network' or 'reflexive' society – a society of cosmopolitan networks, pluralist systems of power, and diverse experiences of inequality – suggests that when we speak about Compassionate Cities we are really talking about compassionate societies.

Compassionate Cities are not literally about cities, high- or low-density living, or the rural–urban divide, but *communities* and how communities of any sort might care for those in end-of-life circumstances – those actually dying, those living with life-threatening illness and those living with loss.

The nature of modern communities has evolved dramatically in the last half century. These reflexive changes to the way people now see themselves demands that we move toward building complementary models to direct service provision responses to care, including end-of-life care. Community development, participatory politics, local and international partnerships, and models of spirituality that reflect these changes in population and religious imagination are crucial to the building of care in the compassionate society. These must begin and be sustainable at the local level and so the language of 'cities' remains appropriate to convey that philosophy. The idea of the Compassionate City is merely a taxonomic legacy of public health ideas that recognize the intimate relations between public and private, and local and global. These social and political tensions have been the foundations for a public health approach towards disease and they are equally relevant to the human experience of death and loss.

The development of Compassionate Cities as a new public health policy is also recognition of past and contemporary deficiencies in those policies. The universality of death and loss has not been recognized as a driving and shaping experience in human communities. This is ironic given the pivotal role these experiences play in current understandings of risk, solidarity, inequality, the politics of inclusion and reflexivity. The ontological foundations of these concepts in political economy and sociology are rightly traced to their ultimate anxieties and symbolic references to death and loss.

As a set of concepts and policies, Compassionate Cities is a necessary correction to contemporary public health theory and practice. It is the shape and substance of a 'third-wave' public health that must come if we are to truly free ourselves of a mundane physical idea of health and well-being. If we are to promote a seamless idea and social practices around well-being and justice – beyond the old categories of 'welfare' and 'health' – we need to embrace concepts and practices that transcend them. Compassion is one third-wave public health ideal that is capable of meeting that challenge.

A Compassionate City approach to end-of-life care is also recognition that such care includes, but goes beyond, palliative and bereavement care. Compassionate Cities require that palliative and bereavement care be recognized and supported in its vital clinical and social mission, but also that these direct service approaches require political and financial support to move beyond them. Public health functions and roles in these professional fields are in their infancy. Lack of recognition by public health of their end-of-life work, however clinically understood, merely retards the valuable progress made by some of them in this area.

A compassionate society is one that has an end-of-life care that recognizes and values both clinical and public health approaches to health care and end-of-life care. It is also one where clinicians and community workers work together for the mutual benefit of each other and the community they serve. Their mutual role is to provide care when the community cannot, and at all times to enhance the inherent abilities of a community to perform that care within the political and social constraints of its resources and vision. The theory of Compassionate Cities is an outline of what is possible to aspire to in such a vision.

Chapter 6

Threats to Compassionate Cities

Even with the best will in the world, the implementation and sustainability of Compassionate Cities will face serious problems. Compassionate Cities face threats to their existence and support from the usual threats that affect any healthy community programme – disease, accidents and warfare, as well as social and physical environmental disturbances. All these affect the health and safety of any community but they also produce the burden of mortality and loss in those communities. However, compassionate communities face additional threats beyond the simple facts of these burdens. In this chapter I want to describe the key challenges and threats to Compassionate Cities that go beyond a community's death and loss toll.

In the first section I will summarize the main threats to Healthy Cities, which also apply to Compassionate Cities. Most of these threats arise from problems of the physical and social environment and are well summarized in the existing public health literature. But threats to Compassionate Cities – to their acceptance as health policies and their sustainability as models of community – come largely from the social, political and intellectual environments of today's modern cultures. These threats are: professional and medical dominance; the gentrification of death and loss; corporate managerialism; economic rationalism, also known as laissez-faire economics; the philosophical conservatism towards new ideas; the media reticence towards death and loss; general taboos around death; and multicultural taboos on the subject of death and loss.

Other matters that threaten implementation and operation of Compassionate Cities include racism and xenophobia; identity politics; secular humanism and scepticism; and the generally unrecognized problem of the apathy of public health movements in matters to do with death and loss. A review of these problems is essential in appreciating the special challenges that lie ahead when attempting to develop Compassionate City policies, remembering that these particular policies make death and loss central to its concerns. Being forewarned is being forearmed.

Threats to Healthy Cities

Baum (1998) gives an excellent summary of the everyday threats that Healthy Cities face. Most of these threats come from the social and physical environment. Climate and atmospheric changes lead to concerns, threats, and actual morbidity and mortality from rising sea levels, affects of global warming, droughts and heatwaves, and declining water and air quality.

Among the social problems that affect the physical environment are urbanization, our dependence on the motor vehicle, chemical and nuclear pollution in general from industries and transport structures but also from disasters that affect wide geographical areas such as Chernobyl, Bhopal or the Asian Tsunami. Also associated with this urbanization are problems such as violence, armed conflict, poverty and the resurgence of infectious diseases. For areas such as Asia or Africa this problem of the resurgence of infectious diseases is highlighted by the devastating economic, social and medical consequences of AIDS, and this problem, in turn, is exacerbated by problems of national debt for countries in this area.

These problems, from rising sea levels to rising levels of poverty or civil wars, do more than simply threaten life and limb. The loss of life and the spread of injury, sickness and disability, are the basic images of public health. These images merely introduce us to the *minimum range* of negative social and physical consequences of physical and social systems where human life is poorly valued or protected. Furthermore, these images are among the shallowest consequences that one can describe because they do not describe the emotional and social impacts that would and actually do promote further cycles of illness and death. These threats to health do not describe the threats to compassion embodied in their presence and consequence.

National systems that are permitted to continue to poorly value or expose citizens to major risk or actual harm, all local catastrophes whatever their origin that kill and maim, fail to prevent major experiences of loss. From experiences of bereavement to those of generational loss and dispossession, major disease outbreaks, civil wars, widespread drought and the pollution of drinking water, all these catastrophes and developments can be and have been the engine rooms for mass migration and global refugee movements. The dispossession and loss over homelands through civil or international war, encroaching urbanization, the disappearance of island states because of rising seas, or the pollution of nuclear tests create not only mass illness, disability and death but the seeds of even more of the same through loss and grief.

And if these were not consequences that brought their own sufficiency of morbidity and mortality, as well as their psychological and social ability to regenerate further poor health outcomes, there is one deeper, less obvious threat. The greater the numbers of refugees, the more overwhelmed a nation perceives itself to be by that problem. The more complex the realities of indigenous need, or the more regular are the casualties of war or poverty, the greater the threat to compassion, as this is felt by individuals as well as governments. Compassion fatigue – the term given to staff who work in palliative or bereavement care who gradually feel emotionally depleted and beyond caring – is a real political, cultural and policy risk in local settings that feel the problems of human suffering that have become too large, unimaginable or clearly beyond their resources. In this way, once again, Compassionate Cities policies rely on the foundations of a Healthy Cities programme, and its social and emotional consequences – and in these terms, its successes and failures.

Professional and medical dominance

One of the single greatest challenges to any sound public health approach is the extent to which communities themselves adopt and own that style of health support. Public health initiatives are often described and implemented by health professionals because they often have the expertise and the scientific knowledge of risk and benefit. The requisite skill and knowledge is one of the outstanding benefits of professionalism, and this is as true of botanists as it is of physicians as it is of veterinary scientists.

But there are disadvantages to professionalism and these have been well documented in histories and sociologies of the rise of the professions (see Friedson 1971, North 1972, Willis 1989). 'Paternalism, self-interest, reluctance to share knowledge and inability to work *with* rather than *on* people' are key observations made by Baum (1993: 37). In matters to do with death and dying, professionalization has led to viewing end-of-life care as a series of discreet problems (as opposed to experiences) that can, or even should be, dealt with by professionals rather than families, friends and co-workers. The professionalization of death has led to a gradual deskilling of modern populations from care of the dying, to preparation of the dead body, to burial, and even to moral and social prescriptions for grieving.

Medicalization in particular has led to institutionalizing the dying person, first in acute care settings and later in hospices for the dying. The movement to encourage and support dying people in their environment of choice, frequently their own home, is a recent positive development largely stimulated by the institutionalization tendencies of medical practice in the last 50 years or so. The medical view of death has also contributed to the secular shift of viewing death as a spiritual journey to one that can be understood as simply a set of discreet disease entities in need of control and taming (Aries 1974, Walter 1994: 12).

If public health approaches to end-of-life care are not to mimic the mistakes of professional dominance by simply converting health policies into health services, instead of facilitating an alteration of community settings and relationships to enhance end-of-life care, it must do so along community development principles. A commitment to these principles means a commitment to a partnership undertaking that begins with the self-identification of a community's own needs. It also means working with and through the third sector – the voluntary sector.

Dooris (1999) argues that bureaucratic governance must be challenged by 'bottom-up' participation by community stakeholders such as trade unions, schools, churches and businesses. Finally, local initiatives must also endeavour to see the global issues and implications of their programmes, in theory and in practice. Bereavement should be seen in broader emotional and social kinship to other losses. Programmes to support people coping with living with cancer or HIV must be seen as parallel initiatives to reconciliation with indigenous people or care for refugees. In these ways, professional action must be equated with community action and not simply with services' responses to end-of-life care matters.

Compassionate Cities are not new *services*. They are community members acting towards each other in new and constructive ways to improve their *own* capacity for end-of-life care. Any professional rationalization of these changes into simpler forms of direct service provision is a regressive and important social threat to community empowerment, a threat to the realization of Compassionate City priorities.

The gentrification of death and loss

The rise of professional dominance is not solely due to some conspiracy from one sector of society to dominate the market in one set of social or scientific skills. Professional dominance is not *imposed* on us but rather it is an outcome of a growing social relationship between a growing number of individuals and communities and their need for particular services. If professional dominance is a threat to simple community initiatives because they will challenge and compete with professional services, another side of this problem will be the preference of modern populations to employ services rather than participate in community and personal development of their own latent care skills.

As I have observed in the previous chapter, reflexive modernity produces people who are bound or attracted to each other on the basis of consumer lifestyles rather than simply workplaces. So many people today change their occupation, their workplace and even their work location that few of us have common social experiences of work nowadays. We *are* more likely to maintain our friends at Rotary, the sailing or tennis club, or watch the same TV shows and drive similar cars. These products and lifestyles – these consumerables, so to speak – are the common currency of our mutual social lives. Busy and specialized work lives also mean that we must purchase most of the basics we need (electricity, medical attention, education or sewerage services) AND the luxuries (entertainment, club memberships, legal advice or accountancy services). However, since an increasing number of us are also professionals, professional encounters are increasingly well understood and participatory. There is a growing demand for 'collegial'-style services and not simply services provided without explanation, discussion or input from the person requesting the service. There is also now a major accent on privacy as a value. As populations moved from farmer to labourer to clerk to professional in the twentieth century, and as disposable income increased, families became smaller and housing more private (Walter 1994, Kellehear 2000a). Families became smaller and work-related migration became common. This meant that informal community support fell away and families depended much more on each other.

A small circle of friends, small families, regular work-related movements and a growing tendency to be private created a major need and desire for professional services. These services were time efficient, individualized, private and were based on rational/scientific forms of 'expertise'. In matters to do with dying, death and grief these made contemporary medical and psychological sciences particularly attractive.

In these sociological ways, modern, reflexive and individualizing needs created a diversity of social norms, a desire for privacy (particularly in matters to do with health and sexuality) and a preference for the professional intervention when trouble loomed. Such preferences make community development models appear less rational/scientific, less 'practical' or less 'direct' in effectiveness. This has been an image problem that has also plagued the history of public health itself, and although community measures to lower morbidity and mortality are well documented they are less powerful as practical images than an immunization programme.

Any Healthy City or Compassionate City policy will need to address the challenge of the 'usefulness' problem that often dogs community initiatives because those communities are characterized by populations who have a preference for short, sharp and dramatic interventions by authority figures. Popular prejudice for professional work as against community work, for interventions rather than preventions and for privacy over public involvement will constitute a major threat to community policies such as a Compassionate Cities programme.

Corporate managerialism

Much of our health system is adopting a corporate managerialist ethos (see Rees and Rodley 1995). There are four observations to make about this introduction of corporate values and attitudes into our modern health care systems (Rees 1995). The managerialist ethos is comprised of four simple beliefs. Firstly, there is a belief that effective management can solve most problems. Secondly, practices for the private sector are appropriate for the public sector. Thirdly, government responsibility for health can and should be rolled back. Finally, we can rely on market forces to regulate health care. I will deal with the final point under the heading of 'Economic rationalism' below.

Since many of our contemporary palliative care services are funded by private institutions or governments who embrace corporate management principles, these principles of corporate management are direct threats to any Compassionate Cities policies. First, health services of any kind cannot address major health problems or disease outbreaks if the physical or social settings themselves are not health promoting. Management issues – corporate or otherwise – are irrelevant to the social and political control of serious health impacts from dispossession, global refugee movements, civil war or the universality of death and loss.

A managerial ethos therefore confines the health policy gaze to small institutions and short-term planning and thinking. Clinical services become the only 'real' problem because this is the day-to-day problem affecting the service. Where the problems originate, their prevalence, or their prevention, become secondary or irrelevant problems for management and, as such, these attitudes and values become serious obstacles in persuading health care institutions to participate in non-economical social activities that address these questions.

Overall, corporate management encourages social values of top-down decision-making, institutional self-interest, content-free practice policies and the rollback of government responsibility for health, to make way for private involvement. All these characteristics threaten Compassionate Cities policies, for these policies require opposite types of commitment to grassroots partnerships, interest in communities, and participatory politics that requires substantial knowledge of the specific needs of communities and their lifestyles and values. Finally, as with Healthy Cities policies, Compassionate Cities require more active government involvement and commitment, not less.

In these ways, the value system enshrined in the corporate management of health services, whether these are government-based or private sector services, create a climate and set of practices that discourage community development and public health approaches. More importantly, funding for community initiatives could be difficult to obtain, as could support from health services businesses. A corporatist gaze is fundamentally a money-making gaze – the goal is financial capital not social capital.

Nevertheless, it will be necessary for a Compassionate City policy to link the two to demonstrate, or to argue, the case that a serious commitment to social capital and healthy individual citizenship is in the interests of good corporate citizenship and a modern image of health care. This new blend of commitment and image may have benefits to corporate activities in the health care area, and in these slim ways are of direct self-interest and benefit to them.

Economic rationalism

As Rees (1995) has argued, the corporate ideology of management cannot be divorced from conservative economic policies such as economic rationalism, or what is otherwise referred to as laissez-faire or free-market economic philosophy. In this view of the world, economic activity should occur with minimal controls and the survival of the fittest will be ensured. Inefficient practices, poor quality products and incompetent management will be swept away with competition. Irrespective of arguments about the value of this economic philosophy for the business world, its application and relevance to the public sector is questionable (Carroll and Manne 1992).

A market-forces ideology applied to health and welfare services is particularly misguided because this field is not a social and economic amalgam of potential winners and losers, providing one kind of service to one kind of clientele. Non-profit organizations abound in this area, as do other agencies where profit is marginal to the main goal of service provision where no other service provision exists. Since most of these services are dedicated to serving the physically and socially vulnerable, a market-forces approach will be detrimental to most providers and their clients.

Moreover, many health and welfare activities do not have profit or efficiency as their main operating goals. Some services and activities exist because current market-based services cannot be justified for their populations. Chief among these are services and activities for people in rural or remote regions, specialist support services for the homeless, indigenous peoples or people with rare medical conditions. Even in areas of high population and with widely shared physical or social disadvantage, not all populations can pay for services at profit-making margins.

Other health and safety programmes are new, untested or are of indirect but certain value to the people who value them, e.g. children's safety house programmes, neighbourhood crime-watch programmes, or grief and sex education in schools. Funding for these programmes, often government funding, occurs because they will NOT be profit making but their benefits are of interest or have been demonstrated. The economic benefits may be obvious but these will often be indirect ones. The economic benefits will be in cost savings because of their preventive long-term role in disease or crime control rather than profits from supplying products or direct services.

Education, community development or facilitative roles are frequently not profit making, and this is a key reason why they are used by governments in their health and welfare programmes. All these roles are, and will be, central to any Healthy or Compassionate City action policy. They will be central for two important reasons. Firstly, rationalization about market demand or justification for funding are essentially reactive comments rather than proactive, leadership responses to the health and safety of communities. Waiting for the community demand for preventive measures around illness prevention or safety assumes that the problem must come before the response. This is a dangerous and contradictory view of prevention. It may be a sound financial response but it is not a compassionate public health one.

Secondly, cost-effectiveness is not simply about profits. Harm prevention IS cost prevention. It is a long-term investment for any government with a view to the long-term future and health of their nation. Public health is a set of rational/scientific principles whose economic effectiveness is well demonstrated, but only if one recognizes that poverty, dispossession, rampant disease, political instability, and the uncontrolled presence of death and loss are bad for business. Conversely, a forward-thinking, economic approach to health and end-of-life care is one that recognizes the social and economic value of public health and compassion. But for some business and government leaders this will be news, and news of dubious value to them. Clear and regular replies to these critics and detractors will need to be available to deal with this growing threat, especially from cash-strapped governments.

Philosophical conservatism toward new ideas

As I have already outlined above, when rehearsing my concerns about professional dominance, we live in a time when, despite the heroic and effective history of public health, health is viewed as the professional's domain. In this way, we exercise our academic and health policy discussions in a context of a contemporary paradigm that sees most of our understanding about power, agency and effectiveness as expressions of professional control. We are used to viewing public health services as government-led programmes to control tobacco use, lessen road accidents, discourage domestic violence, encourage condom use or set the legal age for drinking and sexual encounters.

Recently, death and dying have been assumed to be the province of professional care, and frequently that professional care has been identified with medical care. Palliative care and the so-called euthanasia debate around the world are excellent examples of how complex social and cultural matters to do with dying have become identified with the medical profession. The popular association of cancer with hospice and palliative care has undoubtedly contributed to that link. However, the linking of the medical profession with suicide can only be achieved by implying that there are important psychiatric dimensions to the problem of wanting to die (a highly debatable notion) or of linking that desire with another – to be assisted in the task by a physician.

Nevertheless, this identification of death and dying matters with professional care means that any policy vision which encourages the community to take responsibility for the care of its dying and grieving inhabitants may be subject to significant resistance and derision. This is a common fate of ideas that appear paradoxical to the broader received wisdom.

Schopenhauer (1942) warns that anger and pique is the usual reaction towards new ideas by those who are guardians of the old ones. An obstinate stand will be made against it for as long as possible. After anger, a new idea might be met by a wall of silence, the desire to simply ignore not only the new set of ideas but, in so doing, being dismissive of their presence or growing acceptance. All new ideas are slow to be accepted and late in being appreciated. They will generally be opposed by the more dominant paradigm; in this case, those that give pride of place to the professions and their direct services. If the new ideas are finally accepted they will then be subject to 'competitive praising', by which Schopenhauer (1942: 83) means the second prize next to having the original idea will be being seen to have a 'correct appreciation of it'.

Kuhn (1962) also warns of this problem. He observes that when a science is faced with a severe and prolonged anomaly – in this case the failure to articulate and support a social vision of care of the dying and bereaved – the dominant science will NOT renounce the paradigm. Instead, the science in question will develop ad hoc modifications to protect the current theory to eliminate apparent conflicts. This is well illustrated by current palliative care policies that delegate social and community approaches to care to certain occupations, e.g. social workers who reinterpret community care as community based care. But Kuhn makes a crucial sociological point about changing paradigms.

When paradigms change, the world changes with them. It is important to remember that the problem of developing public health models of end-of-life care will not (in theory or principle) fundamentally change or threaten the original vision of hospice and palliative care but rather the current professionalized interpretation of that care. That version of palliative care may be the major challenge for Compassionate Cities policies that hope to enlist hospice and palliative care workers.

Media reticence

There is no shortage of death reportage in the media (Kearl 1989). Television and newsprint are replete with stories about death. However, what passes for death is frequently merely violence. Murder, disasters and car accidents are chief among the headlines. These events are also quite pictorial and make attention-grabbing visual footage for TV or newspapers.

The bereavement left by these events on their survivors is frequently dramatic and characterized by the expected high emotion of people who have only just learned of their tragic news. Death and loss is literally sensational. It is entertainment.

Living with a life-threatening illness or living with loss is frequently a less 'newsworthy' story, although this does occasionally get media coverage. Films have regularly made these situations into features and it can be argued that 'dying' is a genre film in many respects from *Love Story* and *The Shadow Box* to *Steel Magnolias* and *Terms of Endearment*. Famous portrayals of bereavement are exemplified by *Ghost* and *Truly, Madly, Deeply* among others. The problem with these portrayals is they are often made watchable by the violence or humour integral to the script, or by the following they attract for the film stars they portray in leading roles. The ordinariness of dying and loss is difficult to find in modern film.

Some years ago, when I wanted to write a weekly column on the search for meaning in death and loss for a daily newspaper in my city, the editor informed me that although 'death was a very specialized' topic area they did cover it well in their newspaper. When we reviewed that coverage together we found that most of this 'coverage of death and dying' was abstract or dramatic, and did not reflect the experiences of ageing, dying and loss for most of the community. Although in this instance the newspaper in question did offer me a brief but regular place in their paper, the point of my example is to note the resistance. I doubt I would have been successful in my bid had I not argued my case hard, was a person of high academic status and had talked to an editor willing to engage in a debate about his own views about this subject in the first place. How easily could my bid have fallen on deaf ears.

In the same way that minority groups – ethnic, gendered or sexual minorities – often *feel* they are unimportant and marginal because they do not see images of themselves in the popular media, the same experience applies to the dying and bereaved. When the media does not reflect back the experiences of those living with loss or serious illness people gain the unhelpful impression that their experiences are not important, or are devalued and marginal. But this is not true. Death and loss are universal, and as long as these experiences remain privatized and individualized rather than public and shared we learn about these matters with a significant degree of difficulty. The realities of death and loss feel like they are unshared personal problems instead of mainstream problems and experiences for all of us.

As long as death and loss appear in newspapers and TV programmes in the context of 'problems' and 'tragedies', our understanding of these will be coloured by these terms and concepts. Even positive ideas about living with life-threatening illness, ageing or loss will not be understood as ordinary and multidimensional experiences with complex needs if these experiences have no media representation. In that context, we will continue with an unbalanced emphasis on the need for 'counsellors' in death-related events instead of the surety, safety and continuity of friends, family and co-workers.

Until newspapers have a regular section on compassionate issues – at least as regularly as the sports page, or the lifestyle lift-outs – matters to do with cultural, existential and physical endings will remain largely hidden, embarrassing and decontextualised, and therefore distorted. Such reticence from the media will threaten, if not the actual support for Compassionate City policies, then its ongoing acknowledgement and value.

Death denial, taboos or revival?

There has been long debate about whether industrial societies, particularly in the West, are death-denying societies (Kellehear 1984). Walter (1991, 1994) has even argued that we may be entering a period when interest in death, far from being taboo, may be experiencing something of a 'revival'. Much of this debate is academic, that is to say, a debate concerned with how accurate these descriptors are for a broad range of social conduct such as reluctance by medical staff to speak about death, the cryogenics move- ment or the widespread use of euphemisms when talking about death. Since 'denial' is linked to psychiatric explanations for normal, social behaviour there are clearly problems in resorting to this style of explanation. 'Taboo' is a more anthropological and hence cultural explanation for what is clearly a cultural matter, and the term 'revival' has the same epistemological advan- tage. However, the more specific practical issue – in terms of policy-making – is not whether 'our' societies place taboos on death or whether 'we' are experiencing some kind of revival of interest but *who* views death as taboo or of interest.

No doubt there may be a case for arguing that *some* groups in society are denying death, or rather, some groups in society are denying other group meanings about death. The cryogenic interest groups, who believe that the deceased can be unfrozen and brought back from death when a cure for the condition that originally killed them is found, deny the death that many religious believers adhere to – survival of bodily death in a supernatural realm. Religious adherents who believe in personal survival in an afterlife are examples of death-denial to secular humanists who believe we are merely biological creatures of limited lifespan. Biology, they will argue, is conterminous with life. There is no spirit or soul.

And while funeral workers, hospice, palliative care or bereavement care professionals may have no problem talking about death, dying and loss, the same is not always true of others. There are social difficulties around talk- ing and even reflecting about death. Many people do find discussion of these matters awkward, upsetting or morbid, and do so for a diversity of personal and social reasons. The so-called 'revival' of death may be limited to certain professional circles, some interested audiences, some age groups, or some people with particular experiences and needs. Many others do not share those needs, experiences or circumstances and will resist community strategies that encourage them to draw their attention to these end-of-life matters.

There are three observations to make about these potential obstacles to an open discussion or interactional experiences about death and loss. Firstly, no one should be forced or coerced into discussions or interactional experiences that are personally unpleasant or aversive to them. There is much in Compassionate Cities policies that targets other matters beyond the specific issue of death and dying – addressing the needs of the aged, indigenous reconciliation, helping to accommodate the needs of homeless or geographically disadvantaged, popularizing a community's storytellers or religious traditions.

Secondly, whatever one's personal aversion may be around death and loss, there needs to be a basic recognition that these experiences *are* in fact universal and that important community policies and actions need to be put in place to address these for *those for whom these matters are important*. Either this is agreed to in principle or a needs survey of some description is undertaken to establish the depth, diversity and prevalence of these needs.

Finally, an aversion to topics such as death, mental illness, sex or violence is itself frequently the result of personal and/or community fear and ignorance, and may itself be a barometer for the wider need for more information. Often when I have worked with groups of people with serious cancer the topic of death and dying is initially unpopular, even resisted. Evaluations after the group programmes have finished nearly always reveal that the group discussions about those topics were among the most popular, and this is commonly accompanied by expressions of initial fear and later relief. There are some individuals and groups who undoubtedly need to deny the topic of death any entry into their minds and hearts. For many more, that resistance is not a denial but a taboo based on negative experiences and information about death and loss. For this wider group, compassionate policies are even more important to support.

Multicultural taboos on death and dying

As discussed above, a Compassionate Cities approach to end-of-life care policy will often entail community discussions about sensitive issues, e.g. of suicide, assisted suicide, experiences of living with a life-threatening illness, and the sexual and social issues that arise from this lifestyle or those decisions. There will be talk and information about death and dying and care of the dying. There will be images of ageing, death and dispossession. There will be a diverse array of needs for community information around bereavement but also other 'social' deaths such as lost homelands or lost memories and identities (dementia).

And the problem with many of these topics in a multicultural society is that not everyone will appreciate explicit talk or images of them. Many indigenous peoples do not wish to see pictorial images of their dead. There are widespread taboos on mentioning the word 'death' or even 'cancer' among groups such as the Greeks, the Chinese or the Japanese. Even within these groups, such taboos are unevenly distributed. A Greek or Chinese background does NOT predict these types of social avoidance, as many people from these backgrounds are not migrants who hold these values but American, Australian or British children whose values are similar to Anglo-Celtic citizens. And just as cultural persistence is not certain in any one family group, even the values and attitudes toward death in a society where tradition warns one to tread warily can be unpredictable, as these matters are often mediated by other influences such as education or age.

But verbal and visual taboos in matters to do with death do NOT mean that these populations do not *communicate* about death. Every society communicates about death. As Armstrong (1987) observed, silence is NOT the opposite of truth. Silence is itself a language, a discourse, that speaks its own message as context gently guides its meaning.

The palliative physician Vafiadis (2001), in his study of medical interactions with Australian-Greek patients, found that talk about death and dying with those whose prognosis was clearly poor needed to go beyond simple 'truth-telling'. Disclosures needed to occur over time. Bad news had to be properly balanced with good news about quality of life management and treatment plans (p 50). News about impending death did not simply come from doctors but also friends and family, at times and in contexts that made personal and social sense to the parties concerned. 'Truth' was not always verbal. Mannerisms, periods of silence, rising medication doses or medical attention or progressive symptoms often told all parties about 'prognosis'.

Finally, one cannot take a nominalist position about 'truth-telling' or death in relation to people who live with any life-threatening condition and the community that supports them. Philosophically, clinically or epidemiologically, the prediction of individual death is not reliable. Sociologically, politically and in policy terms, the communication of matters to do with death and loss are more complex and subtle than the taboo on words can indicate. In fact, a literal view of these matters can mislead and isolate. People who support Compassionate Cities policies make it their business to understand the culturally appropriate means and topics that will allow communication about these verities to the communities that need these supports. Fear of offending, and opposition to any attempt to introduce work and discussion of sensitive topics in politically sensitive social groups, artificially inflates a proper concern for vulnerability, so that it regrettably overtakes the more fundamental observation that suffering is a cross-cultural concern of all peoples. It is a mistake to take too fixed a view of ethnic identity, just as it is to allow cultural anxieties to thwart creative partnerships in addressing the most universal of all human experiences – death and loss.

Racism, xenophobia and cultural reproduction

If the desire not to harm others of social and cultural difference can be a threat to compassionate policies then its opposite – racism and xenophobia – are even greater threats to supportive partnerships. The problem of racism is also a major challenge to preserving a community's storytellers and spiritual traditions, or to addressing the issue of indigenous reconciliation and refugee loss. This problem of racism can take at least three forms: outright racial hatred and vilification; xenophobia – the mistrust and anxiety over any 'outsider' irrespective of origin; and cultural reproduction – the frequently mindless duplication of one's own values, people and social processes without regard or thought for other equally eligible or appropriate choices.

Each of these three expressions of racism threatens the development and implementation of compassionate policies. Racial hatred and vilification is arguably the easier problem to identify and manage, usually because its hostility consists of violence and/or open opposition to the distribution of resources of any kind to the disliked groups. The development and support of local and state laws against racial vilification are important in discouraging and controlling racist acts. Racist attitudes and values are another matter.

Educational approaches have been the key suggestions of anti-racist community strategies (Council of Europe 1995). These strategies have involved anti-racist school education programmes, intercultural understanding opportunities such as festivals, concerts or public lectures, and anti-racist media campaigns. Other strategies include anti-racist and culture-appropriate training for teachers, police and businesses, intercommunity links, and equal opportunity employment practices and laws. All of these strategies and more are crucial in addressing racism and xenophobia, but with respect to death and loss more needs to be done.

The *social and cultural* similarities of the experiences of loss and physical endings need to be made and explored by different communities. This type of exercise will encourage an appreciation of the importance, power and depth of cultural loss, and social alienation, by comparing the emotional and intellectual processes of these experiences with those of facing one's own death or the bereavement experience. Consciousness-raising about everyone's spiritual or religious understanding about dying, death, burial or cremation practices, bereavement, and afterlife beliefs can be facilitated by more publicity, education or experiential opportunity for different localities.

The problem of cultural reproduction is equally a threat to be addressed by any compassionate policies (Jenks 1993). Employment practices, or use of volunteers, trainers or media figures, in the service of implementing anti-racist campaigns that do not themselves reflect the cultural diversity of the population they wish to target is literally a nonsense. Dominant groups, particularly well-educated ones, are extremely adept at reproducing their own racial, gender and class networks, and frequently do so with an impressive array of intellectual rationalization and justification. Women in the workplace know these male habits only too well. But class, age and ethnic patterns of cultural reproduction are not confined to gender circumstances.

In the end, commitment to a concerted and self-conscious attempt to break this cycle of practice is needed not only for the goals of equity and access but also for credibility and success of any attempt to welcome and embrace social difference.

Identity politics

If racism, xenophobia and cultural reproduction are threats to compas-sionate policies from those who are openly hostile or self-absorbed, identity politics is also a threat to those policies from groups who wish to make a virtue of one social difference (Anthias and Yuval-Davis 1992). The organ-ization of groups who collect and work together on the basis of common problems of alienation, discrimination or outright exclusion has been important to the organized challenge and resistance to these matters (Fook 2002). But there are ironies about these forms of organized reaction, which can mitigate against a broader, more inclusive politics that views social dif-ference in multidimensional ways. The following developments illustrate the problem.

Many countries such as the USA, UK or Australia have long broken away from stereotypes and discrimination of others based on country of origin. However, the politics of multiculturalism has, to some extent, replaced one stereotype (country of origin) with another ('ethnic groups', 'blacks' or 'Asians'). These and other recently employed 'cultural categories' tend to assume an 'essentializing' quality in the minds of other people. In other words, these labels perform two functions: (1) rather paradoxically they fail to convey differences by highlighting just one, e.g. colour; and (2) they overidentify certain fixed qualities or characteristics to a group without recognition of the uneven distribution of those qualities in the group being described. In this way, although well intentioned, the labels are unfair.

Blacks are gay or straight, men and women, working or middle class, Christian or Muslim, are representative or not of different generational cohorts. Everyone has *multiple* identities. The links between what we appear to be, what we are, what we do and how we do it are complex because they are shaped by different aspects of our whole identity moment-to-moment. Although an understandable, often appropriate, response to resistance and acceptance by dominant groups, identity politics can exhibit a parochial self-interest. Such groups have been accused of being too inward looking and separatist (Bourne 1987).

In this context, the politics of difference can be overly identified with differences in social and political resources, and not with broader matters of inclusion such as commonalities and universals of human experience. By an uncritical emphasis on struggle and resistance, and on the personal and the sectional interest – of ethnic, class or gender differences – we can unwittingly deepen the divisions between each other by portraying these interests as our total selves.

As Anthias and Yuval-Davis (1992: 194) argue, 'Establishing a system of identity politics as a form of resistance to Eurocentrism, Orientalism and racism fails exactly because its basic assumptions have been formed within a discourse of difference it wants to attack.' Hence the threats to the development and support of compassionate policies from identity politics then come from singular rather than dual strategies of resistance. In this way identity politics can be slow to recognize that overcoming estrangement from dominant groups is not simply about challenging their aversion to difference but also in demonstrating the universal traits and experiential connections we have in common with one another.

A Compassionate City policy must enlist the support of groups that view themselves as marginal in a particular locality. In so doing, the implementation of those policies must tread that fine line, recognizing the importance to those groups of their differences but also encouraging those same groups to advertise their common experiences with others, particularly in matters to do with death and loss. Finally, a compassionate approach to policies about identity and memory in respect to death and loss in war, dispossession, colonialism, or suicide and illness is to appreciate that both identity and memory are *highly selective and socially constructed*.

As Gillis (1994: 4) warns, they can be inscriptive as well as prescriptive, serving particular interests and ideological positions. Public commemoration and memory about beliefs and memory change, as each new generation asks different questions about the same events, experiences or people. There must be recognition of that changeable and complex nature at every point, or religion and history become merely an ideological stick that one group employs to bludgeon another.

Secular humanism and scepticism

Radest (1990: 65) argues that, 'Those for whom reason is the essence of Humanism find spirituality an affront.' I do not want here to argue that organized humanism is a threat to the policies of Compassionate Cities, although these organizations have been active in criticizing organized religion, informal New Age movements and ideas, and parapsychology. Sceptic

organizations and publishing houses have been at the forefront of champi-
oning materialist explanations for mystical experiences such as near-death
experiences and visions (Kellehear 1996). Often their criticism is not without reason or merit and their critical functions as organizations have been
important to providing sound alternatives to superstition, irrationality, false
claims, bogus theories and outright intellectual or social stupidity.

Nevertheless, these organizations – symbolically and sociologically – represent a growing number of well-educated people for whom religion and
the recent academic and popular discourses on spirituality are troublesome.
For people with humanist leanings – those who assume there is no God or
afterlife, and any beliefs about the divine or afterlife such as might exist are
irrelevant – believe that science and reason are the key tools for human
progress and survival. Spiritual issues *may* be valuable but there is wide
disagreement about what that word might mean (see Radest 1990: 49–80).

However, there is no reason why spirituality need be necessarily and
automatically connected to religion (Kellehear 2000b), if by that term we
speak about the meanings people construct to transcend their everyday sufferings. If humanist existentialism is not to be written off as 'religion' there
is no reason to expect that intellectual debates and research, or community
or professional discussion of spiritual matters cannot be culturally inclusive
of the religious and non-religious members of any community.

In palliative care, where spirituality discourses range from the outright
religious (because of the strong presence of Christian groups in this field) to
the aggressively and reactively materialist (Bradshaw 1996), views about
spirituality tend to polarize. But such reactions are simply distorting, and
do not reflect the fruitful personal and social strengths which people may
draw and enjoy from developing attitudes and explanations towards events
and experiences that carry them beyond the certain and concrete forms of
reasoning. This does not automatically lead to the irrational any more than
the desire to be reasonable bestowing a guarantee of it.

Encouraging a community's storytellers and spiritual traditions requires
that community to be tolerant of those traditions. This policy position does
not require that we, as individuals, embrace those traditions if they are not
ours or have no appeal. But it does require that we understand the importance of spiritual beliefs (religious beliefs and non-religious humanist
beliefs) to the task of making sense of the life we have and the sufferings
that we must endure, and transcend.

In this context, religious intolerance must include sceptism and secular
humanism if these beliefs actively oppose the celebration of religious beliefs.
This threat to the celebration of diversity must also include religious sectarianism as part of the problem of identity politics, wherever this exists. But
while we are accustomed to think of religion and ethnicity as potential social
problems, we are less likely to view the less high-profile secular humanism as
a potential source of intolerance. This is not necessarily the case.

Recently my own university proposed a new Bachelor of Pastoral Care degree programme and as this degree underwent its usual scrutiny through various school then faculty then university-wide committees its existence was regularly threatened by humanist assumptions that this was 'religion' sneeking back into the university. This flys in the face of the fact that most people remain committed to religious beliefs in one form or another, the fact that the curriculum was multifaith and the fact that the core skills emphasis was on meaning-making for anyone whatever their beliefs. The university is largely a secular institution, and although its charter is tolerance of all ideas, when religion or any of its cousins appear in its halls, sneers can still be heard in its corridors. Intolerance is no longer simply a religious trait. Compassionate policies may be threatened by humanist kinds of beliefs and prejuduces, apparently because those who champion reason may have this facility desert them at key intervals.

The apathy of public health

One of the most impressive facts about public health is its narrow treatment of death, dying and loss. For the practitioners and policy-makers in the field of public health, death is an event or a threat (Henley and Donovan 1999), not an experience. And while death appears as 'mortality', loss barely rates a mention at all. Articles on Healthy Cities never mention death or dying except as something to avoid or prevent. When the word 'loss' appears it is usually associated with 'loss' of health or physical function. Public health laments inequalities among refugee, indigenous populations or the poor working class, but rarely explores the impact of grief on the health of those populations despite a significant literature establishing this link (Raphael 1986).

The three-volume *Oxford Textbook of Public Health* (Detels et al 1997) explores health maintenance for the frail aged and HIV infection issues, but all but ignores matters to do with death and loss. There are discussions about death certification, rates and 'avoidable' causes of death, and the brief inclusion of palliative care as a topic is merely to note that this is on the opposite end of the public health scale to preventive, curative or restorative medicine. Grief and loss are so ignored as a subject by this public health tome that 'meals on wheels', 'mouth rinses' and 'puffer fish' rate an index entry over their inclusion.

The four-volume *Encyclopedia of Public Health* (Breslow 2002) is also largely silent in these matters. Hospice and palliative care do rate an index entry but these services are viewed as 'last-days' type terminal care (p 1006). Grief is identified with bereavement and this associated with direct service provision by counsellors and hospices rather than any genuinely community based public health strategies (pp 110–11).

Palliative care workers and academics debate the nature and meaning of 'public health' as applied to care of the dying and those living with loss. And while they question its meaning, even existence in palliative care, public health workers seems to believe death and dying to be someone else's problem (Kellehear 1998). Many think that if a public health approach to death and loss were possible that this might be an issue for palliative care or bereavement care workers to take up. This is not only a professional death-avoidance style of thinking and policy-making, it is also a reflection of the shallow connections made by public health between health, identity, and death and loss.

As long as public health theory and policy maintains a position of death-avoidance, and as long as palliative care maintains its clinical course of development, few will take up the public health challenge of engaging the community in the task of its own end-of-life care. And ultimately that end-of-life care will become one of the single greatest challenges of an ageing, mobile, multiculturalist society in the twenty-first century.

If we fear institutionalization at the end of life, if we deplore the ongoing morbidity and mortality of refugee and indigenous peoples, and if we aspire to maintain our own health until the end of life, we require a seamless public health approach to life that is inclusive of death and loss.

That approach, and that challenge, is the promise of a compassionate public health.

Chapter 7

Implementation: making it happen

The central question for all practitioners involved in developing community practices for end-of-life care is how to make Compassionate City policies real. While one may agree with the broad outlines of historical and policy analysis of the current gaps in community participation in end-of-life care, how does one actually begin to practically re-engage community in its own end-of-life care agenda? In other words, what practical steps towards implementation can a person or agency take to develop an approach that can develop a Compassionate City?

The theory and practice literature that addresses those questions is commonly called 'community development', 'community capacity building', 'community work or community action ' literature. Writers in this area provide principles and practices that instruct the reader on the best ways to encourage communities, neighbourhoods or other social networks to invest in their own social welfare and health. Much of the Healthy Cities literature borrows from the concepts and language of community development, and public health writers in this area have also developed their own style and models of what they believe works best.

In this chapter, I will begin with a brief introduction to the idea of 'community development'. I will then describe four general implementation models that readers might find fertile as frameworks for their own plans in implementing Compassionate Cities. These four models are: the Healthy Cities model; the Community Development model; the Community Focused Professional model; and the Unpaid Community Activist model. In reality, all these are variants of a broad class of community development. I separate them out to describe the different emphasis each takes because of the traditions of theory and practice from which each comes. It is also valuable to underline the different approaches that emerge by highlighting WHO (community members or professionals or patient/client groups or local government workers) is doing the community development with WHOM (cross-combination of WHO). The final section of this chapter will end with a brief discussion of the value and methods of evaluation in the practice of community development.

What is community development?

Community development is any set of initiatives designed to develop the social resources of the community in order to enhance its quality of life. This means that community development initiatives may cover a broad range of recreational, health, welfare, educational and workplace dimensions of social life. However, what distinguishes community development initiatives from simply government or business initiatives is that the needs, wants or problems identified are those articulated by a cross-section of the community affected by those needs or problems.

Furthermore, solutions to the newly identified needs or problems are not sought simply in advocating for greater provision of private or government services. Solutions are sought in connecting people and resources together in new or novel ways. Indeed, sometimes the impetus for community initiatives has to do with the limitations or shortcomings of existing social services. For example, police cannot be everywhere at all times so 'safety houses' for children and 'neighbourhood watch' are initiatives developed by neighbourhoods with police to transcend the understandable limitations of a paid surveillance workforce such as the police.

At other times, services may be criticized for shortcomings of their offerings. For example, a clinical service may provide excellent nursing and medical services but little in the way of ongoing social supports. Advocacy and support groups, or community education nights, may all contribute to overcoming those shortcomings by linking vulnerable groups with people in the same situation or by educating the wider community about how they might assist in the plight of particular groups.

All community development initiatives have as their main aim the desire to deepen the quality and extent to which a community may look after its own members. This may come about to enhance existing services, or sometimes to reach beyond the limitations and shortcomings of those services, or even sometimes to create alternative structures of care from existing services. The following models of community development practice illustrate the different ways a Compassionate City programme may be established, as well as how these approaches are connected to different aims, resources, political style, skills and commitment (Table 7.1).

Table 7.1 Models of community development practice

Model	Aim	Role	Politics	Skills	Commitment
Healthy Cities	Policy change	Statutory	Group	Corporate	Part-time
Community Development	Transcend services	Employed	Insider–outsider	Organizational	Full-time
Community Focused Professional	Improve services	Paid activist	Paid insider–insider	Personal	Part-time
Unpaid Community Activist	Create alternatives to services	Voluntary activism	Insider–insider	Political	Full- or part-time

Healthy Cities model

Aim

The main aim of any Healthy Cities programme is to introduce changes in the community to enhance that community's health. This will often require events, information and institutional experiences that bring about attitude and behaviour change, which will lead to the promotion of greater health and safety in the community. In other words, a Healthy Cities programme is a programme of policy and culture change.

Policies that assume that direct health services are the most adequate ways to address health needs, or that those health needs are best identified by 'experts' rather than neighbourhoods and communities, or that health care is best left to state or federal agencies, are all policies requiring change. Underlying such policies are assumptions that point to disempowering health care practices. These policies assume that health needs and supports should be identified and addressed by agencies outside the local community.

The policies also recognize 'expert knowledge' and authority but not local knowledge or experience with health and illness. Finally, these policies assume that a service response to health care needs is a one-size-fits-all one. The recognition of the special roles and value of non-service type interventions and supports – learning and support systems, for example – is inadequate in these types of policy assumptions.

Healthy Cities programmes then are designed to change the above policies and cultural attitudes (in professionals and communities) so that people are able to take greater responsibility for each other's health care. In Compassionate Cities programmes, the aims may mirror these kinds of criticisms and reservations, but additionally focus on matters to do with death, dying and loss. We may also feel that a direct services response, the emphasis on professional knowledge and experience, and a lack of local initiative hampers a community's ability to look after its own people at the end of life. We may feel that palliative care or bereavement policies in our state are inadequate in identifying and addressing all our needs in these areas of life. If our aim is to support a major change to these kinds of policies and values then a Healthy Cities model of action might be attractive.

Role and action emphasis

Healthy Cities programmes frequently advocate involvement with a statutory authority as soon as possible. In other words, one of the first things to do if you want to establish a Healthy City (or Compassionate City) programme is to enlist the support of local government. Tsouros (1990) argues that the first step is to participate in the statutory mechanisms of decision-making. This does NOT mean one needs to get elected to council but it does mean that one must convince the local council of the worth of greater involvement in health care (or end-of-life care).

Fryer (1988) lobbied the local Labour Party in the UK, through the health trade union, until he gained a political commitment to form a Health Liaison Committee and Health Working Party. These were pressure groups within the Labour Party and these acted as further pressure groups to influence council of the merits of a Healthy City programme in the city of Oxford. Ashton et al (1986) also argued for the need to establish a Healthy City Committee as a decision-making committee of council.

Less directly political, at least initially, is Dahl's suggestion of creating 'community round tables' – forums where anyone can come, literally to a large table – and discuss with others from the same community the problems and solutions in health or end-of-life care as they all see it. At these round tables people are then able to sort out 'needs' from 'wants', set priorities and plan the initial steps for political and social action. These actions might include lobbying the local council for some statutory involvement.

Different Healthy City practitioners and theorists advocate different ways to involve the community. Dahl recommends round-table discussions but Fryer, for example, advocates public consultation through newsletters and public forums. Other writers advocate less direct ways of seeking to understand a community's needs, such as conducting a population survey of needs or holding a community conference or consultation with non-government organizations and peak bodies. Within each of the different suggestions for initial action a common theme seems to be that the political style is corporate and group driven.

Political style

There is an assumption in Healthy City programmes that the best way to achieve change is: (1) to use the local statutory powers of council as a lever for change; (2) to form a coalition of interests, from the different sectors of a neighbourhood if not a community, as this is the most effective way to influence people in that neighbourhood; and (3) work as soon as possible with *formal* organization. This political style has several merits.

Firstly, organization means a shared division of labour and multiple personalities, social positions and ideas to draw upon. This enhances problem-solving ability and broadens the initial resources base of the programme. Secondly, such committees may enlist important members of the community who represent powerful agencies within the community, or are themselves powerful and influential figures in their own community. This can be important for credibility and change. Thirdly, local government involvement can mean the development of important and sustainable gains through local policy development. This means that sustainability is not entirely dependent on a particular generation of enthusiasts for change because the momentum might be sustained through the institutional pressures of a policy document. That document, in turn, may have council staff supporting its ongoing operation.

There are disadvantages of such organizations. Firstly, by enlisting important community power brokers one tends to favour powerful interest groups over those who are important culturally but marginal politically. Representativeness can become a problem. The risk of reproducing attitudes and values about health care or end-of-life care may be a considerable risk. Secondly, the personal challenge of setting up a formal organization can be a disincentive, or simply discouraging, for individuals who are committed to Compassionate Cities but whose talents for social change may lie in working directly with small community groups and not local business people, professionals or councillors. This formal organizational political style may not suit their personal style, or even that of the community for whom they wish to work and represent!

Skills emphasis

Healthy City programmes emphasize a number of skills relevant to the political style of their preferred community development approach. These are principally lobbying and organizational skills. It is important to be able to be confident enough to phone or arrange meetings with important community power brokers from business and local government, as well as the public sector health area. The personal ability to communicate well, to persuade and to inspire will be helpful, if not crucial, to this political style of community development.

Tsouros (1990) emphasizes the importance of developing pressure groups, of engaging the voluntary services, and developing advocacy and media skills. Other skills discussed by Ashton et al (1986) include the need to develop a funding development strategy – to fund educational/informational programmes, to employ staff or to create and maintain a minimum data set about the morbidity and mortality profile of a community. Writing skills and an ability to network and enlist the support of diverse agencies, such as radio stations, art galleries or local schools, will be important. Organizational and management skills will be crucial to the success of any Compassionate Cities approach employing this particular political style. However, as I mentioned, the committee-style leadership, and partnerships with local government, will ensure that there is always a possibility of employing people with the right skills or of having such people on the actual steering or management committee.

In these ways, the skills emphasis is *corporate* – favouring skills that attract the mainstream elements within a community – and making the case that a Healthy or Compassionate Cities programme is one that will 'value-add' to the community's solid stock of health and social services. The idea is to create robust communities that are supported by their key leaders and social settings to enhance support, safety and health to a level that goes beyond the sufficiency of current services.

Commitment

Finally, the Healthy City approach – because it emphasizes committee organization, government partnership and funding development – often means that actual commitment of time and involvement can be part-time for the individual. Often a good division of labour, the use of specific-purpose employees or the fact that funding does not cover anyone full-time, means that any one person must be involved only on a part-time basis. For professionals who wish to be involved or to lead a Compassionate City programme, but who must also juggle a clinical workload, this can be an ideal commitment, which *does not* mean less actual work may get performed because other members, agencies or staff may continue the work when they are unable to do so.

Community development model

Aim

Most community development models of practice do not necessarily aim to create policy or cultural change. Some do actually have that aim but most other community development initiatives are designed to *extend or transcend current service offerings*. The chief aim is to 'capacity build', to help communities to address their needs in cooperative as well as formal direct service ways.

Many services in welfare or health recognize that direct services to communities, such as counselling, medical or social services, have their limitations in addressing broader issues such as drug and alcohol use, domestic violence, or diabetes or heart disease. To tackle some of these issues more effectively, service agencies attempt to develop ways that make information and support structures more accessible, or practices more readily adopted. Social contexts are often crucial to people's ability to access, learn or accept, and most of these relate to workplaces or recreational sites, and activities and experiences conducted in the positive environment of friends, family or workmates.

The recognition of the importance of these sites and relationships to the health and well-being of people are the key reasons why many community health and welfare agencies actually employ a task-specific worker with the official designation of 'community development worker' or 'community worker'. At other times community work may be the primary task of a social worker or health-promotion worker. Whatever the employment choices made by agencies, such appointments reflect the fact that addressing human need must employ both direct service and community approaches to well-being, and so the community development approach becomes an employed- or paid-worker response to this broader philosophic recognition.

Role and action emphasis

Logically then, community development models of practice nearly always employ a worker or two specifically for this role. Whether specifically trained as a community development worker, or whether community development is part of a broader training in social work or public health, the role is diverse and dependent upon the specific brief of the agency and their target population. Unlike the Healthy Cities approach there is no necessary requirement to enlist the support of the local city council. Indeed, the local council may actually be one of those agencies that employ community workers for their specific purposes of youth work, drug and alcohol use, health promotion with sex workers or the homeless, for example.

The most important observation to make about the employed community development worker is that they are always nearly provided a special-purpose brief by their employing agency. If your bereavement, palliative care or community health agency has a commitment to the development of a Compassionate Cities programme AND you have the necessary funding, you may choose simply to employ a community development worker. This worker can then lead and manage the programme under the governance of your agency.

According to Kenny (1999) and Homan (1999), such workers will be employed to empower others in the community, to problem-solve their anxieties or resistance to supporting their neighbours, and to develop simple cooperative starting points for the programme. They will coordinate and connect people with one another and will employ outreach methods – visiting people, organizing public meetings, enlisting volunteers, talking to the media – to create a grass-roots campaign to develop a Compassionate Cities programme.

Cox et al (1984) list several important roles for the paid community development worker. These include organizing a community coalition of interested groups and individuals; funding development; political lobbying; running meetings, networking and community participation; providing community education and being involved in radio, TV, Internet and print media. Ife (1995) argues that community development workers might also have research skills, be prepared for and experienced in public speaking; running groups; be able to resolve or manage conflict; advocate; and motivate and enthuse others.

But Ife (1995: 227) is also quick to point out that every community and every community worker is different, and each brings different challenges and talents to each other. There are few recipes for a good community development worker other than being a lateral thinker, problem-solver and communicator.

Political style

Unlike a Healthy Cities political style, which is based upon group-driven benevolence, the political style of employed community development workers tends to be an individually driven activism. The job is to raise community awareness and participation in their own health or well-being, but to do so in ways that complement and enhance the mission of the employer agency. The community development worker is ultimately responsible to a single agency and its mission. This may be more or less constraining than being responsible to a Compassionate City committee of the local council and hence to elected officials.

Furthermore, many community development workers are not necessarily from the communities in which they are employed to work. Youth workers are not always young themselves, or from similar social classes to those people. Community development workers with drug users or the homeless are not always ex-users or formerly homeless people. Even more simply, workers who are employed to work in a particular suburb are not usually, either in the past or the present, residents of that community. It is from this assumption that many community development texts describe a political style that is best characterized as an 'insider–outsider' relationship.

Community development workers are frequently well meaning and experienced outsiders who are trained to assist the community to help itself. As the community becomes adept and confident in its new-found roles and activities, insiders take over the roles and activities formerly organized or initiated by the outsider, i.e. the community development worker. Homan (1999) describes this as the sliding balance between social action (by a well-meaning outsider) and actual community development (escalating insider control and activity). The first phase of any 'community development' is really attributable to the social actions of the community development worker. But as his or her actions stimulate and succeed to enroll the interest of the community, genuine community actions and controls begin to exert themselves and prevail. Ideally, this can lead to the gradual withdrawal of the paid worker, as the goals of community self-care actually become operational.

Skills emphasis

Although many of the same skills that are required for a Healthy Cities programme are also necessary for any community development programme the emphasis is slightly different. Working to persuade local government or power brokers in the community does throw significant emphasis on leadership and organizational credentials. But because most community development workers work with special populations the skills emphasis is more highly personal. The ability to be credible, and to convey empathy and rapport with those populations is crucial in enlisting the trust and cooperation of those particular populations.

It may not be necessary at all to go anywhere near a statutory authority in any shape or form. Most of the work a paid community development worker might do is inside the actual community itself, and/or in specific community settings such as schools, workplaces or churches. It is very important that the paid community development worker has the personal skills or experience to initiate a broad range of projects because that worker may need to rely on only those skills rather than draw on a working committee or co-participants with similar skill levels and experience.

The choice of community worker then becomes an extremely important appointment process, as personal credibility with the target population is balanced with formal and personal skills at the actual task of community development. In these ways, the skill emphasis can be characterized as one of advocacy and critical reform. We begin with an acknowledgement that a direct service approach may be insufficient for the task and challenge of community health or well-being. At the same time, it may well also become necessary to see the world from the point of view of that community. That role reversal may position the community development worker as critic, and lead to tensions between the agency and the community at best and potential conflict at worst. Nevertheless, this is the skills tightrope that the paid community development worker walks.

Commitment

The single greatest advantage that a paid community development worker has – and the agency that employs such a person – is that commitment to the development of a Compassionate City approach will be full-time. Whatever the shortcomings, an employee whose full-time job it is to develop the programme has the advantage of providing continuity and constant application to the many tasks involved in gaining interest and enlisting the support of others.

It is also the case that many people can only provide partial support with other work to which they are dedicated. A paid worker allows consistent and accessible contact and coordination for a wide group of part-time but equally committed members of a Compassionate City consortium, coalition or committee.

Community focused professional model

Ife (1995) singles out several community development roles that might not be so designated but can perform many community development functions. One of these roles, which is relevant to a Compassionate City approach is the community focused professional and the other role is the unpaid community activist. I will address the first here and the second role in the next section.

Aim

If the agency you work for has little additional funds to employ a full-time community development worker but remains interested and committed to the idea of community development then the obvious alternative is to per-mit one or several of its professionals (or volunteers) to do this work. Most of the time the community development will be done by one interested member of the team and this will be the 'community focused professional'. The main aim of encouraging and supporting one or more members of the team to develop a Compassionate City programme will often be to improve and complement the existing service offerings.

There will be recognition that a direct service approach to the health and well-being of the community can be enhanced and improved by comple-menting these services with community work. This will add to the existing 'service offerings' rather than attempt to transcend or overtake them in any way. Just as some services offer face-to-face specialist consultations of one sort or another, and perhaps also offer group work and community educa-tion, community development initiatives will be seen as an *additional serv-ice strategy* that will round out the agency's overall approach to health or end-of-life care.

Community development in this context will be employed to allow the agency to participate in community activities, and to encourage community members to participate in the life and mission of the service itself. Such community development work, in palliative care for example, may start with expanding the role of volunteers to include encouraging the involvement of schools or trade unions in the activities of the palliative care service. In a complementary turn of that relationship, the service may also organize meetings or media events where these same members of the community get together to design ways that they might care for people living with loss at school or the workplace.

Whatever the actual initiatives, the aim is always to improve the role of the service in the context of the agencies desire to work *with* the community rather than work *on* the community. Community development is always a genuine attempt to create compassionate collaborations that go beyond mere clinical services.

Role and action emphasis

Basically, the community focused professional as a paid activist may come from a diversity of backgrounds. They may have a community development background, experience or credentials and will have some good initial ideas about how to proceed. Those professionals familiar with Healthy City programmes may want to take their ideas about Compassionate Cities to city hall immediately and lobby council for a coalition or committee. Others who already live in a Healthy City may wish to approach council to broaden the brief of their existing Healthy City programme. Others still may wish for a more low-key approach that may be more considerate and realistic of the fractional time allocation these professionals may have set aside for these tasks.

For those with little or no community development background it will be important to familiarize oneself with the basic literature of community development, health promotion, Healthy Cities programmes and health-promoting palliative care. From that initial study one can develop some early ideas about how to proceed, and what modest projects are possible within the time, talents and interests of the community focused professional.

The paid activist, like the full-time employed role, is one that is constrained by the mission and ideology of the agency. This does not mean that the community development programmes that these kinds of workers adopt are of less value than those developed by Healthy City committees. It might mean, however, that unlike those committees, all actions by the employed community development worker or community focused professional will reflect on the agency itself, and this can act as a brake for some creative and controversial initiatives.

Political style

The political style of the community focused professional then is similar to that of the employed community development worker – both are frequently outsiders who must be aware that they are on someone else's payroll and are ultimately responsible to that employer. One may not immediately think that this could be constraining for a Compassionate City programme but it can be.

Consider the community committee that decides to support their local voluntary euthanasia society and the community focused professional is employed by a Catholic palliative care service. Or consider the agency whose funding comes largely from government contracts. What if the community focused professional is part of a compassionate education campaign that leads to conflict with that government about the state of local indigenous health or welfare?

Similar to the employed community development worker, the community focused professional is also an individual driven by activism. This has two strengths and problems. First, there is often a genuine commitment to see things from the point of view of the community that they are attempting to serve. This commitment is as it should be, and permits the worker to view and act employing a practice framework different to the one he or she usually employs. That framework enhances the worker's ability to understand the problems and challenges faced by that community from their point of view. However, this can also inadvertently lead to criticism and potential conflict with the service and its mission. It can also lead to what some anthropologist's describe as 'going native', i.e. taking sides with the community! This is always a risk and an ethical dilemma for any committed professional who views matters from a social justice point of view rather than in terms of loyalties.

Secondly, as an outsider to a community the community development worker or community focused professional is able to see things that insiders take for granted, and are therefore unable to see disentangled from their own local politics or infighting. Outsiders can bring a fresh perspective to long-standing problems (as well as naivety) but are more easily dismissed because of their outsider status or new ideas. Equally, paid outsiders, acting alone, can be accused of having a vested agency interest in certain programmes rather than the welfare of the programme or community for their own sake.

A commitment to a Compassionate City programme is laudable, but being paid to initiate that programme leaves one vulnerable to distrust by individuals and communities who have been used, abused or who have been failed in some way by 'professionals'. The political style of the individual paid activist is a freer role and political style to that of a committee-driven initiative, but it is also one that must be much more reflective and cautious because of that freedom.

Skills emphasis

The skills emphasis is not significantly different to those required by any community development worker, but clearly time and previous training and experience are the ruling constraints. All the usual skills of public speaking, research, media work, organizing ability and networking and so on that is required of the community development worker is also required of the community focused professional. Often it is time rather than interest or skill that eclipses all other issues. In that context, it remains a good resource idea to begin any Compassionate City programme with an organizing or steering committee to help drive the programme, if only because the committee will have additional assistance for the community focused professional.

There are many ways to establish that initial committee. One can invite from key areas of the community, e.g. schools, trade unions, churches, non-government organizations, local councils, emergency services, law enforcement agencies and the local palliative or bereavement services. One can invite key political figures within a community as power brokers, decision-makers and influences within the community. Or one can simply advertise over print, radio or TV media for expressions of interest from anyone interested in such a programme. For the community focused professional it will be important to decide on what particular policies and how much you want to achieve in a certain time frame, and how best to achieve these goals. One can then decide about whom might best be recruited from what parts of the community to help you facilitate those policies.

Commitment

The community focused professional is commonly only able to devote a part of his or her time to community work. This is an important constraint but it also highlights one of the first priorities that a community focused professional might set for themselves – funding and resource development. One of the key contributions or activities that any business, council or participating agency might make is some time, personnel or funds for administrative assistance, or time release for the community focused professional.

One of the advantages of the Healthy City approach is that council may be persuaded to take on the administrative support of the programme as one of its contributions to the programme. Another possibility is to apply for funding from local and state governments, or from private endowments and charities, for some support for the compassionate community activities. A part-time commitment makes these kinds of initiatives crucial to the initial momentum and success.

Unpaid community activist model

You may not be reading this book as a health care professional. You could be simply anyone interested in end-of-life issues, from bereavement to aged care to the politics and psychology of loss. You may not be part of a health care agency of any sort. You may not be particularly involved in direct practice or policy development. You may, however, be someone who has significant personal experience in loss and grief; someone who may be dissatisfied with current health service responses to bereavement care, palliative care, indigenous health care, aged care or many other areas of life affected by life-threatening illness, ageing and loss. Your experiences might just drive you to become an unpaid community activist.

Aim

In this role you might wish to create alternatives to service offerings. You may be critical of professional involvement or distrusting of government and bureaucratic responses to loss and serious illness. You would not be the first to hold these kinds of criticisms or reservations, and the lack of participatory relationships in professional relationships generate an increasing number of like-minded critical people every year. You might see in a Compassionate Cities programme the opportunity to create an alternative politics of help, a grass-roots response to end-of-life care that can be created and driven by people with common experiences in the diverse array of events that is illness and loss.

Compassionate Cities ideas can be driven by people who have first-hand experience of serious illness and loss, and who are critical of mainstream clinical responses to these. Your aim might also be to use a Compassionate Cities programme as a basis for engaging direct services in a reform agenda, and dialogue, that may lead services to take partnerships with community as central to their design and operation.

The aims of the unpaid activist then are to: (1) create alternative practices that strengthen community supports by facilitating those most affected by death and loss to become leaders and educators for other members of their community; (2) to create an ongoing dialogue with direct services to broaden their accountability to those they desire to serve; and (3) to create partnerships with all sectors of the community that are initiated by the community rather than those defined and initiated by professionals.

Role and action emphasis

The unpaid community activist is likely to be the most political activist of all the practice models so far reviewed. Often the unpaid activist is passionate about their cause because they are aggrieved or simply because they keenly feel a gap not currently addressed by services. Media work will be crucial in gaining support and resources for their Compassionate City programme. The art of persuasion and good communication skills will also be important, both for the task of media work and also to persuade some key social institutions to join you.

Since your only role to date may be as a volunteer, or as a member of a community support group or advocacy society, the ability to inspire others to help you develop a Compassionate Cities programme will be crucial. You are not going to be able to employ a community development worker nor is your employer likely to release you for part of your work hours to be an activist in some area not related to your usual work.

Crucial to your success is the ability to bring others together and to bring those people together with passion equal or approximate to your own. Once again a coalition of some sort will be needed to help with the work responsibilities that come with lobbying and with persuading organizations that you do not normally have a relationship with to cooperate with you. It's one thing for the local city council to listen to a representative of the local palliative care agency; it is quite another for them to listen to someone advocating a Compassionate City programme who is the local carpenter or high-school pupil. But the local high-school pupil or carpenter has just as much right to be interested in and to initiate a Compassionate City programme as any health care professional. That is the fundamental meaning of ANY community programme – that citizens from any walk of life can and should initiate them, with or without the 'blessing' of professionals.

Political style

There will be a temptation to take an adversarial political style. There are good traditions of this in the gay and lesbian community, but also the indigenous communities around the world. It is not for me to weigh the benefits and disadvantages of such a style, only to recognize that an adversarial position has been useful whatever its drawbacks. It is particularly useful when diplomacy and networking have failed or when positioned (however willingly or reluctantly) by groups who vehemently oppose your bid for resources for whatever reason.

That said, there are also good grounds for believing that partnerships are more difficult to obtain when the request comes aggressively, resentfully or at the end of a long tirade of criticism. This appears to be a cross-cultural feature of social relations. As they say in ballroom dancing, 'lead with your best foot'. The main political style should be to employ one's network to *expand* its allies and friends. This is best done diplomatically, with intelligence and forbearance.

In this way, the clever political style of the unpaid activist may be characterized as *insider–insider* politics. Unlike the paid community development worker who has two 'masters' (the community and the employer), and who is most likely not a member of the community they wish to serve, the unpaid activist is a member of the community and has only one loyalty. There will be no gradual withdrawal of commitment, only changes in the role as the tasks become greater and more multiple.

Skills emphasis

The skills most likely to be embraced in this political style are those designed to bring about significant change. They may be adversarial without being overtly aggressive because they are designed to bring social justice and support for the broader aim of end-of-life care. And the passion for that drive may come from a difficult personal experience. Personal experience can be a disadvantage but it can also provide depth of understanding and great commitment where a lack of personal experience can lead to ignorance and maltreatment or mistreatment.

Two key skills will be important – media work and lobbying ability. If these are not readily available to you then your coalition of interested people should include some that are experienced or confident in these areas. Criticism and calls for reform have that much more power when they become public calls over the airwaves, and this in turn makes those calls more pressing when they appear at the door of local or state government politicians. Remember, community development is not direct service provision. Community programmes, whether they are Healthy or Compassionate Cities programmes, or sexual health programmes, are political programmes of change. How widespread and effective they are in bringing true social change to the neighbourhood, your state or the country as a whole depends very much on the impact you make in your public and political communications.

Commitment

Unpaid community activists may be full-time or part-time. As a full-time activist they can be extremely effective because the only limitation of their community development work is time and personal commitment. Full-time activists have plenty of both.

The other resource that unpaid activists often have is other people who share their criticism or personal experience. Joining with others with like sentiments and experiences creates powerful lobbies that few employer groups can rival with paid community development workers or well-meaning professionals. In this way, characterizing commitment into full-time or part-time only barely suggests the energy and creativity that unpaid activists can bring to tasks such as a Compassionate City programme.

Box 8 Common activities in community development

Political lobbying	Public meetings	Public speaking
Media interviews	Popular writing	Funding development
Networking	Educational activities	Research
Public consultation	Organizing	Management
Self-help groups	Persuasion	Communicating
Evaluation	Conflict resolution	Developing support
Collective action	Making allies	Devolving power
Submissions	Petitions	Criticism (giving and receiving)

Evaluation: are you really improving end-of-life care?

Evaluations are methods you employ to assess whether your social programmes are working or not. They can be as simple as surveying people before and after a programme to see whether there has been a positive, negative or no impact on them. Most books on community development advocate the importance of evaluating the social programmes generated by that development. There are good reasons behind this advocacy.

Why evaluate?

Firstly, evaluations are excellent ways to assess effectiveness in an organized and credible way. Why do something if you don't know whether it works? Evaluation is the way to get an answer. Secondly, evaluation helps you build political and social support. In other words, evaluations that indicate that you are being effective help convince other people that the programmes are worth doing. Thirdly, evaluations are useful ways to obtain feedback for your future planning. It is quite rare that you will get a programme exactly right the very first time, and feedback from the people exposed to a programme will help you adjust and modify the programme for greater effectiveness in the future.

Fourthly, regular feedback improves your practice. Feedback builds practice wisdom. Length of time doing something does not give you anything more than empty experience – it is feedback that converts experience into learning, insight and expertise. Fifthly, feedback from evaluations helps you refine policy as well as practice. Some of the Compassionate City policies you have read here may not suit your particular community and may need extension, omission or modification. You may need to develop new, additional policies that apply to your community. Evaluations from your programmes may give you strong research-based feedback indicating those needs and changes.

Sixthly, evaluations provide a basis for understanding further community need and also what things you need to do further than you are currently. Occasionally you might believe, on the basis of initial-needs assessment through open public forums or surveys, that you have assessed a community's needs on a particular subject well. Evaluations of a community programme may be the first indication that you have overlooked something. Finally, regular, diverse and imaginative evaluations improve your research skills. This can lead to growing independence from consultants or the need to pay for and rely on outside advice. Regular evaluations make you thoughtful about how to obtain the most reliable and valid feedback for your programmes, and lead to growing confidence that your results are the best you can obtain with current social research methods.

Which methods?

So which methods might you employ for evaluation? Evaluation method books fill substantial space in most academic libraries but most of them are not a difficult read. Discard those that are difficult and browse ones that you can understand to get started. Some people naturally prefer surveys with some simple statistical analysis that they can perform on their personal computer. Others prefer more qualitative, narrative-based feedback mechanisms. The important point to make here is that one must recognize the difference between obtaining subjective 'happy-sheet' results and more convincing indicators of actual change. If you provide people with 'feedback' sheets asking them about what they *thought* they gained from a programme you will most likely gain an impression of their immediate reactions. If, however, you ask them to respond to a case scenario before and after a programme you are more likely to be able to observe a measurable difference, which may be above and beyond the participant's feelings about their enjoyment or otherwise of the programme.

Whatever methods you employ it is a good idea to 'benchmark' a state of play and attempt to assess movement away from that position. That benchmark could be an attitude towards some topic, people or social issue. The benchmark could be an ability or usual response to a social situation. For example, one could ask people what their first words and response would be to a work colleague who reports the death of his or her child. After a programme designed to heighten people's awareness of the bereavement experiences one can ask the same people their response once again.

One may use surveys and interviews as well as observations. The observations can be participant or non-participant. One can employ 'action research' methods where both the research topic and the methods are chosen by those within the programme. One can choose reflective methods where people are asked to unpack their assumptions behind a critical incident and to explore other ways of responding and interpreting. You can employ unobtrusive methods using existing personal and public records, examining media representations, photos or social and physical spaces that people use in their daily lives and how these change.

Social experiments are also useful ways to gauge change. Dropping addressed envelopes in the street at different locations to observe how many are actually found and posted back to the address. You can measure this again over several months as an indicator of growing or lessening social capital (or trust) in the community. And finally you can employ self-reports by key stakeholders to assess whether, objective or not, those key stakeholders actually *believe* that things are improving in their community because of the presence and application of Compassionate City policies.

Credibility or getability?

Evaluating is only partly about the credibility of your claims about programme effectiveness. It is also about your ability to obtain resources in a competitive environment. There will always be detractors towards any social justice programme. On both sides of politics, conservatives and more liberal thinkers will exist and they will differ about the adequacy of any programme or policy. Social capital and social justice are controversial and ambiguous topics on which to obtain broad agreement. Sound research results help gain your programme support but they will never guarantee it. But the mere fact that you evaluate will assist you in your political claims about accountability, and therefore in your bid for resources against those who would attempt to quickly discredit you. That is simply the politics of resource allocation.

When your results are in, always remember that for some people good results are never quite good enough. The levels of significance are always too weak; the methods you employed somewhat flawed, or very flawed; the sample atypical or too small for generalization. Even when the results are beyond scientific dispute they may already be 'too old' because 'things have already changed in that community'. And a good result can be an equally good reason to halt the programme because the job has clearly 'been done'. Positively good evaluations are a necessary but not sufficient device to persuade others of the worth of your work. This is not a reason to be dispirited, but it is important not to be naïve about the importance of credible research methods and results. We must acknowledge the wider context of all science, and all efforts towards social justice and social compassion – the politics of social life itself.

Simple or not so simple?

The Australian social worker Ife (1995: 227–9) cautions against what he calls 'the use of cookbook' approaches to community development. He wisely warns against the idea that community development is an orderly, linear process because it is often not. Community development is frequently a messy, back and forth process. He warns that every community and every community development worker is different – every community has different social features and every person has different talents and interests.

But for readers for whom the phrase 'community development' is new, some basic ideas about what actions are involved in this form of social and political activity IS important. The models outlined in this chapter are designed to give the reader some broad, if academic, models of possible practice that they as individuals or as employed agency workers may emulate in some approximate way in their own attempts to create a Compassionate City where they live or work.

It is important to acknowledge the important role of personal differences and equally important differences in communities, so that one does not measure success by some artificial and context-free yardstick. But at the same time 'cookbooks' are often spurned by those who have the luxury of no longer needing them. For those of us who have never cooked before such introductory exegeses open the door to new worlds. If community development ideas excite and tempt you away from direct service ideas about end-of-life care then read all the 'cookbooks' you can lay your hands on. Use everything you've got to help us use everything we've got in our communities.

Chapter 8

Action strategies

In the previous chapter I described some basic implementation suggestions on how to begin to establish a Compassionate City. You can do this alone as an activist or professional, or you can get started by forming coalitions with other professionals and/or local government. As in everything else in life there are advantages and disadvantages to each approach. But once you have decided to commence a Compassionate City programme, alone or with others, your attention will quickly turn to the question of what kinds of activities will you actually attempt to promote?

Clearly, a wise and *participatory* approach is to attempt to establish what the *community itself* wishes to see established by way of compassionate programmes. This will be an essential ongoing communication challenge for anyone attempting to develop a Compassionate City strategy in his or her community. However, not everyone will know what 'Compassionate Cities' are, or indeed is able or experienced enough to know what activities might be attempted in that name. Some suggestions or example ideas can form the basis of community ideas. This chapter is written in the spirit of prompting and proferring.

In this chapter I will make a broad range of action suggestions that can easily help materialize or support compassionate policy ideas. The following suggestions are NOT designed to be taken as the best or most ideal way of supporting Compassionate City policies. These activities are offered as a guide and illustration of what some communities or activists might consider by way of public health actions that encourage communities to take a greater role in the care of their people living with life-threatening illness and loss. Obviously many other suggestions are possible and relevant. A peruse through works such as New Society (1988), Putter (1997), Mayo (2000) and similar works can inspire members of any community or profession to think about 'grass-roots initiatives' from drop-in centres to community singing groups. Below, I offer 25 suggestions to stimulate readers to think of their own possibilities, or indeed even to experiment with some of these suggestions in their own communities.

There is no 'magic' number of community initiatives. Clearly one initiative is a bit of a poor showing. Conversely, attempting to juggle 30 or 40 community initiatives, all facilitated and organized through one agency or local government community committee, may be completely unrealistic. The number will depend on the size of community and professional commitment and time resources. Some activities will attract wide attention and participation, while others will be confined to small groups or localities. A combination of both types of action strategies is optimal for success.

Poster campaign

A poster campaign is an excellent way of raising awareness about loss. Posters have been invaluable in health-promotion campaigns for the prevention of sexually transmissible diseases, drink-driving, school bullying and numerous undesirable behaviours. The basic prevention problem with respect to loss is the sometimes problematic nature of other people's responses towards the bereaved.

Chief among the problems encountered by bereaved people are the inability of other people to make appropriate and comforting social responses; to provide a sustainable level of social support; and to underestimate the importance of the loss to the bereaved. Some of these responses are due to the tendency to see appropriate social responses in terms of talk rather than listening; to view grief as akin to influenza, dramatic but short-lived; and to trivialize grief in relationships that do not occupy mainstream social status, such as animal companions, divorced partners, country of origin, elderly parents and so on.

Posters can be developed by an expert committee in partnership with community members, and distributed into a diverse range of workplaces, schools and recreational areas such as clubs, hotels and recreational societies. They can be placed prominently but unobtrusively in phone booths, toilets, near vending machines, tearooms and lounges. They need to be short and practical. They can be humorous or serious, but they should always be practical and to the point. Poster information should be easy to remember. I supply two examples.

Box 9 **Comforting a grieving person**

- Remember – it's not so much what you SAY but how well you LISTEN
- Do not make the suggestion that they 'will get over it': they may not but will need support during periods of the most intense feelings of sorrow

- Do not discourage or be embarrassed by crying. Just wait, listen and support with a comforting hand. Offer to get drinks or tissues
- Do not make assumptions about the nature of OTHER people's relationships. People grieve over the deaths of dogs or cats. Deaths of friends may have greater impact than deaths of relatives. The death of former spouses or distant friends may evoke powerful feelings of loss
- Be yourself but allow the grieving person to express their own thoughts and feelings about their loss
- Be prepared to provide time and listening opportunities for their loss for a long time – not simply days or weeks but months and perhaps years
- If silence makes you uncomfortable, encourage the grieving person to tell you about the relationship they have lost
- After the funeral do make sure that your attention does not drop away. Call or offer to help with small tasks such as shopping. Invite them for company but do not pressure them to accept these offers
- Be aware of special anniversaries as times for remembrance and return of intense sorrow, e.g. Christmas, wedding anniversaries, birthdays or anniversaries of the death. Be around or call or make the offer

At your school, place of worship or workplace, ensure that notices such as these are prominently displayed with other notices for health services, including those for spiritual or psychological counselling. These should ALWAYS be displayed, not simply at times of crisis or tragedy.

Box 10 Pet loss

- Strong feelings of sadness over the death of an animal companion are NORMAL. All the usual emotions of grief can be present
- There are many people who are embarrassed or who trivialize the experience of loss over an animal companion. These are usually innocent but ignorant people. Ignore them
- Choose supportive, animal-loving friends to talk to. Your local vet can also be a useful resource person. He or she can provide sound advice or support to you or suggest others who may provide similar support

- Don't be afraid to use a counsellor if you feel you need that extra bit of support. Many people avail themselves of this service and do find it useful
- It is *not* unusual to feel the presence, or to occasionally even see, your dead. Many people have reported these experiences. This is not a sign of mental illness. There is much we do not understand about the nature of death, sorrow and the human mind. Consider yourself lucky, not mad
- Don't feel badly if burial of your animal companion in your back-yard is not possible. There are other ways to memorialize. You can bury their collar or playthings in your yard. You can donate unused food and old toys, or make a financial contribution to animal welfare organizations
- Where practical, always respect the wishes of your children and never force them to be present during euthanasia or burial if they do not want to. In the same spirit, do not keep them away if they want to attend either
- It is NOT betrayal to choose another animal companion soon. Nothing can replace your former companion but nurturing a new friend can ease pain and foster hope through the formation of a new relationship and future

Trivial pursuit nights

Trivial pursuit nights are very popular community activities. They can be organized by local service and sporting clubs, and they are fun activities for staff, parents and children at school too. The topics one may employ for such a night are limitless but for raising awareness about loss, for example, a night exploring world consolation words and rites will be thought-provoking and informative. It can stimulate people's ideas about how they might creatively respond to another's grief by designing their own personal response from the cultural information about other people's rites and words of consolation (see for example Adamolekun 1999).

Obviously it will be important to provide teams or individuals attending the night with a broad range of literature on this topic before they attend. Alternatively, trivial pursuit cards can be made up with multiple choice answers on them. Professionals in grief and palliative care can assist in the compilation of the answers as well as the design for the questions themselves.

Positive grieving art exhibition

Although schools and communities have sometimes encouraged artistic expression of loss – among their own, the indigenous communities or among special groups of children – they seldom emphasize the positive experiences of grief. An art exhibition encouraging schools or communities to design art to give expression to the positive aspects of grieving will be important to bringing emotional, social and spiritual balance to our understanding and experience of grief.

People continue to have relationships with their dead through dreams, ambitions or actual visions of them. Greater personal sensitivity and social empathy frequently comes to those who know loss intimately. Political activism, social advocacy and funding development are all positive human legacies that are directly derived from personal grief (Kellehear 2002). Personal courage and much public civic vision comes from personal tragedy and these, among other social, personal and spiritual qualities, can be highlighted in community arts exhibitions.

Annual emergencies services round table

We often forget those who deal with sudden death on an everyday basis in the community. These are our paramedics, police, firefighters and other emergency workers. They live in our community and endure great stresses and grief in their daily work. It is important that such workers are encouraged to recognize the special difficulties of their mission, and that they are regularly encouraged to seek out sustainable ways of supporting each other in the pursuit of their important community work.

An annual 'round table' is a discussion forum for these emergency workers in the local community designed for them to discuss organizational ways that recognize and support these special stresses and satisfactions of their work. Although counselling services and supervision are important ways to recognize and support personal problems, the experience of grief is far more than mere problems. Collegiality, informal supports, public and peer recognition, and accessibility of ordinary social information about loss and its diverse expression can provide a preventative approach to problems of stress, isolation and grief in this kind of work, and removes the problem of any incidental social stigma.

As members of the community who routinely deal with traumatic and violent death, an annual discussion forum to exchange information on the latest information, services and practice models about these matters, along with informal networking and support opportunities, will be an invaluable community initiative. This can offer a community the opportunity to support those who support them all year round.

Public forum on compassion and loss

A public forum on compassion and loss is actually a good way to commence a Compassionate City programme. In this forum one can place on
display, for public comment and discussion, the four central concepts of
Compassionate Cities as well as their nine defining characteristics. This
type of public display and its accompanying discussion forum can enable
professionals and activists to gauge public interest, as well as acting as a
forum for feedback and suggestions.

Most importantly, such forums can generate volunteers and fellow travellers that have interest, time and commitment to these ideas. A coalition of
these interests can be formed from the initial interest that such a forum
might generate. These forums can also be important networking opportunities, as well as preparing a community for a follow-up needs/wants
survey.

But even if this is not to be an *initial* action strategy, a public forum on
compassion and loss is a useful public health device. A forum can raise
awareness and educate people about the links between compassion and
loss, different types of loss, the needs of people living with life-threatening
illness in their own community, and the personal, social and spiritual issues
surrounding all these connections. Such forums can also generate important
support and publicity about what the community is trying to do with
respect to its own *self-care* around death and loss, and that fact alone can
generate greater participation for other later initiatives.

A public forum can also be a useful venue for a public debate about compassionate care – the debaters can be from local business and the professions or even the local schools. These can be thought-provoking
accompaniments and prompts to other activities in the forum.

Review of local policy and planning

Most local governments have policies or planning models for public health,
disasters and community services, but what about compassionate policies
that support those living with life-threatening illness and loss? Of those
governments with policies to support loss or serious illness, how many of
these are simply policies that support the bereaved or those with cancer?
Local councils need to be asked – and asked publicly – what these policies
are. A review of current policies needs to explore the central concepts of
Compassionate Cities and to compare the adequacy of current policies in
that light.

For example, a bereavement support strategy is not a comprehensive
strategy to support loss. Some idea of the burden of living with loss and the
needs of those living with this experience should be gained. A public forum,
a needs survey or an unobtrusive exploration of the social and historical

profile of the community will provide strong indicators of the experiences of loss in that community.

It is important that, among other action strategies, lobbying the local government for a review of their policies is an action that contributes towards the goal of sustainability of compassionate programmes. If the local government gets behind these values and policies they have a greater chance of being inherited and adopted by successive generations of locals.

Annual short story competition

One important way of raising people's awareness of the burden of loss and care in the community is to advertise and support a local short story competition. The runners-up or the best half-dozen pieces can be published in the local newspaper as well as the final winner. These are excellent ways for readers to gain an understanding of the details of caring for those with dementia, cancer, AIDS or motor neuron disease. It can give poignant detail and insight into people's daily experiences with loss. It can be a great and substantial basis for community empathy and support.

But beyond simply raising awareness, the appearance of several stories a year about the experiences of people with serious illness, those caring for them or those living with loss also permits those people to see themselves in the public representations of the media itself. These are important ways that communities can reflect about their own identities and the diversity of experience within its own networks.

Finally, a local short story competition is a normalizing and comforting way for people to express themselves and their own experiences. Winning or losing is a minor outcome to encouraging people to reflect on their own experiences through the act of writing and then reading that experience back to themselves. This can play an important personal role in self-understanding and a local writing competition targeting a compassionate topic can help facilitate these personal processes widely in the community – a valuable health-promotion strategy.

Annual peacetime Remembrance Day

Although in many countries war veterans have an annual day to march and remember their dead, few places have an annual peacetime Remembrance Day. There is no reason why this should remain so. A peacetime Remembrance Day can be held the day after or before the annual veteran's Remembrance Day and can be a march to a particular memorial site chosen by popular suggestion. Marching groups can walk together holding photos of their loved ones and may carry banners representing different suburbs, ethnic groups, ages or experiences of loss.

It is important that the annual peacetime Remembrance Day truly represents a diversity of experiences of endings and loss. Women who have lost a baby during pregnancy may march alongside indigenous peoples mourning the loss of their land, traditions and ancestors to violent dispossession. People who have lost family or friends in car accidents may march alongside those who have lost colleagues in workplace accidents.

Such marches serve to usefully remind people that death and loss occur every year among them and that, at least for some, the cause of death may be preventable or avoidable. In that context, peacetime Remembrance Days can deliver important public health messages for preventable deaths. On the other hand, these days can also help a community to embrace all losses and to seek or develop important social empathy towards groups for which they may have had only very limited understanding.

Walk-a-mile-with-me Week

A useful community experience is to set aside one week every year to assist people to understand the joys and burden of care. Aged care facilities might open their doors to the local service and sporting clubs and ask members to accompany and assist staff in caring for the elderly for one week.

Alternatively, workplaces might sponsor a different lunchtime talk from members of the local carers association, motor neuron disease association or dementia care association. These speakers and many others from carers groups and organizations might be welcomed into the workplace for a lunchtime to speak about the diversity of experiences in caring for someone with a serious illness. The local peak organization for grief or palliative care might also receive such invitations too.

Newspapers might also be encouraged to run a special feature that week on carers, living with serious illness, living with loss, and the typical day of the emergency worker or palliative care professional. Once again, apart from raising awareness and sensitivity to the issues themselves such special weeks increase community solidarity and social capital.

Mortality network

If Walk-a-mile-with-me Week has no appeal then a 'mortality network' of experts, from funeral, grief or palliative care, can be organized and advertised to visit schools, workplaces and service or sporting clubs to speak to people about particular aspects of death, dying or loss. These people can supply valuable information about the facts of death and loss, but they can also facilitate useful discussion about matters that often create apprehension or frank anxiety around death and loss. They can provide comfort as well as information, generate interest and respect, as well as humour and support.

Death and loss will never be normalized as long as we treat both the topics and the professionals in death and loss as outside our interests and needs. Funeral or bereavement care will be accessed by most of us, unlike occupational health and safety officers, council public health officers or CPR training. If any of these former occupations or skills is considered necessary by you how much more important are the more certain verities and skills during the life course. A mortality network gives ordinary people the opportunity to demystify aspects of death, dying and loss that they may not otherwise have unless they have a direct personal encounter. A mortality network enhances a community's prevention and early intervention abilities by employing its own professionals before an urgent time of need.

The social meaning of suicide

Many suicide prevention programmes emphasize early detection of character or mood changes. However, an equally valuable and complementary prevention strategy is to work with family and friends of suicides to describe the personal, social and spiritual impact of suicide on those left behind. Many families who have experienced the suicide of one of their own speak of the stigma and isolation they frequently feel because one of their family has committed suicide (Fraser 1997). There is a great need for public education in this area.

A public campaign about the aftermath of suicide can raise community awareness, combat ignorance and may act as another prevention influence on those contemplating suicide. There is a great anxiety within professional communities and media that public discussion of suicide might increase its incidence. But there is no evidence that a concerted, deliberate increased and widespread discussion of this topic may not be useful to everyone concerned. NOT speaking about suicide has its own psychological and social morbidity. Certainly shame, stigma and blame are experiences that are protected by ignorance and hidden by community silence. We must balance the needs of those who are contemplating suicide with those who must live out the consequences.

Information packages for workplaces, churches and recreational clubs – simply one-page leaflets distributed once a year – can be important community information. Such information can also be blended into Walk-a-mile-with-me Weeks or annual peacetime Remembrance Days.

Mobile death education unit

Similar to conventional public health programmes worldwide, many public health education campaigns appeal to white-collar workers or people who like to read. Furthermore, it is difficult to ask schools to take on additional education programmes on top of their current curricula and extra-curricula activities and programmes. Every social development has a tendency to target schools and additional resources can be difficult to find.

In this context, a mobile death education unit could be useful to develop and fund as a community action strategy. A mobile home unit or even an estate car (a station-wagon) could be used for one or two education officers to visit schools and factories to impart practical information about death, dying and loss. The exact type of information imparted by this service needs to be identified and agreed upon, but this could range from information for carers of those seriously ill or impaired to social information on how to respond to those who have recently become bereaved. Other types of information that could be useful are will-making, funeral arranging or the physical and psychological effects of grief.

The unit may carry poster displays, photographs and research information both in summary and plain-English form. The unit can also act as a mobile library of books and video material. Films and documentaries on caring, living with life-threatening illness or living with loss can be shown at lunchtimes to interested audiences. Games, group exercises and role-plays can be facilitated by the mobile unit, as well as referrals and educational information about local human services.

Neighbourhood watch programmes

Neighbourhood watch programmes have enjoyed much publicity and considerable success as crime-prevention strategies. The idea is that whole neighbourhoods are encouraged to watch over the property of their neighbours and to report suspicious behaviour to the police, quickly and early. This principle of community involvement and responsibility in the safety and well-being of others can easily be applied to the health and well-being of others.

Building on existing crime-watch programmes, neighbours can be encouraged to observe and reflect on the health, age-frailty or sudden death of their neighbours and their animal companions. Offers to feed pets while neighbours are away, or in respite care, are examples. A simple but regular offer of help after bereavement can be helpful. An invitation to a social occasion at your home can be a compassionate neighbourly response to the stresses of care if you are both able to problem-solve a short-time replacement for the carer. If this is a difficult idea – and for many it will be because people who work and who have families are usually busy – then a monthly roster for this special kind of neighbourhood watch might be a way to distribute the task.

An inclusive annual veteran's Remembrance Day

An important obstacle to compassion, indeed all forms of social empathy, is the ability to identify with the troubles of another person or group.

Compassion and empathy are easy tasks if you are a member of the group experiencing the trouble. In this way, there is great camaraderie, and strength, in shared troubles. But as one moves away from groups that you easily identify with, empathy becomes conditional and difficult. With despised groups, empathy is often absent or merely intellectual. The limits to compassion are so often the limits to personal experience. In these ways, Remembrance Days are so often inward looking and non-inclusive. Such sorrows readily breed criticism and resentment toward people who are believed to have been responsible in some way – however real or abstract – for the deaths of those they love.

However, blame, resentment, discrimination and hatred are enemies of compassion. Such attitudes fly in the face of the facts of the universality of loss. In war, both sides lose loved ones. WHY that happened is the problem of historical and political analysis and not the subject of community mourning. The community recognition that the early death of loved ones should be preventable should be an important universal message of compassion and peace for all annual Remembrance Days. Japanese and Americans should be able to march side-by-side in remembering their dead. Death and rape should occupy the memories of all those who participated in war as important losses for all sides.

An ongoing community programme of reconciliation with former enemies around the universal social, personal and spiritual problem of loss during national days of remembrance is a worthy and therapeutic public health task, as well as a contribution to the prevention of further wars.

School and workplace plans for death and loss

Many schools but few workplaces have plans to deal with the sudden death of staff, students and workers. Where such plans do not exist they should be developed. What company responses towards families can be expected by employees if they die suddenly? These should include descriptions of benefits and entitlements but also interpersonal responses and services from the company. Beyond counselling, what interpersonal responses can be expected from a school when one of its staff or students suddenly dies? How does a workplace or school deal with any of its members who are bereaved? What leave, financial services or personal provisions can be made? Written plans for these compassionate issues should be routine.

An audit of such plans in the local area's schools and workplaces will be a major community initiative, which will create major discussion about what kind of community we all wish to live and work in. The idea that compassion can be more than a private response to troubles can receive a practical illustration in the writing and implementation of new local policies in this area. Plans can be compared and contrasted, and differences in planned responses debated and discussed as a community issue.

This leadership in community action can be led by local government or from funeral, grief or palliative care agencies. Churches can encourage and lead by initiating similar audits in their funded organizations and services. A commitment to education in death and loss should be part of any school and workplace plans, and not just ideas and suggestions for direct support in time of need. Remember, compassion is more than action in time of need – it must include prevention and early intervention, and this places education at the centre of any social response.

Investigating the links between loss and crime

We often think of crime as creating loss. Losses of property and of life itself are common dimensions of crime. But how much of crime itself is a response to personal losses in an individual life? I do not necessarily refer here to organized crime, i.e. crime that has major sociological and economical links. However, some violent crimes, crimes of social disorder such as drunkenness, some drug addiction, some aggressive conduct and other destructive behaviour may have personal roots in earlier experiences of emotional loss. A screening programme in partnership with local police, the judicial system and welfare services may be able to identify such links, and commence community or professional support services for these people, particularly first offenders.

Offenders who have been sexually abused may find it useful to link up with others who have endured such experiences, to listen and engage with the later experiences and choices made by these people. Social responses are created by a combination of circumstances and personal choices, and it is often unclear where one begins and the other ends. Sometimes only a discussion with those who know your own type of loss intimately can give you insight into your own decisions and leanings.

Such a programme can easily become a professional service without major input from the community. There can be no doubt that professional services here will help, but a crucial role for that service will be to forge the links with community groups who represent different types of loss and crises. Without those linkages there is no community development of responsibility towards its own. This particular suggestion might also complement the annual emergency services round-table initiative as an additional way to create partnerships with community.

'Speak My Language (of Experience)' programmes

Three or four times a year eight people can gather together, not to debate, but to compare and contrast their experiences of living with a life-threatening illness or living with loss. The eight people are divided into two groups of four. From this division the parties can vary, four men and four women discuss living with cancer, or four men and four women discuss caring for a partner living with dementia, or four Christians speak about living with loss with four Muslims living with loss, or four indigenous people speak about their experiences of loss with four refugees. These can be open public forums or they might be organized by local churches or service clubs for their own members. These groups can also be arranged by local schools or health services for their own staff or students.

These special discussion groups should occur every year and with people from a different combination of compassionate circumstances. The idea is to select an experience – caring or coping – and choose two groups on the basis of social or cultural difference. There will be no shortage of groups to encourage participating and after a couple of years there will be a need to repeat sessions for new audiences.

These group discussions of comparing and contrasting allow community members to learn about the differences within their own community but also the similarities of experience. The forums may act as an important source of critical understanding about the diversity of experience and identity within a community, and can be important in supporting and sustaining social empathy.

Finally, 'Speak My Language' programmes permit a wide variety of community participation because few people do not have their own care or cope experiences with serious illness or loss. Such programmes can create a broader camaraderie and support within the community by encouraging new networks based on existential/circumstantial identification. These can lead to new friendships and support networks that are health promoting and sustainable.

Palliative care for beginners

This is a partnership programme run by palliative care professionals WITH members of the community who have experience caring for seriously ill or elderly family or friends. Together this partnership can run a one- or two-day workshop on end-of-life care. Professional knowledge can complement, question or underpin lay knowledge and vice versa.

Initially such programmes should target those who are currently caring, bearing in mind that some respite care will need to be arranged for such carers to attend the workshop. Both professionals and community participants conducting the programme will need to make these arrangements, or take responsibility for the care itself. The advertising should inform potentially interested parties accordingly.

Later these programmes can encourage other community members to participate. Alternatively, separate programmes for those who have little or no experience with end-of-life care can be conducted concurrently if resources permit. Those programmes can and should be advertised at workplaces, schools, churches, and service and sporting clubs. As demographic changes to the age profile of most industrial societies head toward the elderly, more and more people will become interested in the challenges that many of them will have to face, particularly with elderly parents. These workshops will attract interest.

An important health-promotion dimension to these workshops will not only be the care issues – social, physical, psychological and spiritual – for the person who is ill or elderly but also the care issues for carers themselves. How do carers – professional and lay – look after themselves? What are the health challenges for them?

'Volumes of Compassion' book club

Book clubs are increasingly popular today. They are an enjoyable way of meeting new people with similar interests while being able to keep up with new and interesting literature in a favoured area. Easy to start, many neighbourhoods start their own book clubs with work, church or recreational networks. They begin with three or four friends and then friends invite other friends. Sometimes a service club or church organizes these book clubs and several groups coexist side-by-side.

The idea is that a particular book is chosen, ordered and then read by everyone in the group at the same time, over an agreed period. They then come together at regular intervals to discuss the contents of the book, debating and reflecting on the finer points of the argument or story. Once finished another book is chosen and the whole process begins again.

In a 'Volumes of Compassion' book club, books that cover all the areas of Compassionate Cities policy vision are relevant: death, dying, loss, dispossession, abuse, as well as spiritual books with existential reflections and arguments, world religions, humanism as well as parapsychology. And of course this literature will contain volumes of poetry, fiction and art that covers these topics.

The ultimate aim of the 'Volumes of Compassion' book club are to encourage people who have no time, energy or desire to participate in more public activities, such as festivals, writing competitions or public forums, to devote some of their recreational time to reflection on compassionate issues. People who are private in their recreational pursuits or who work alone and don't often hear about or are offered other Compassionate City programmes may find these type of activities more unobtrusive and suitable for their lifestyle.

The role of loss in the social history of the local community

Every history employs a framework to organize the story of how things seem the way they are. Local histories are one important way that local communities (and nations) rationalize or understand their identity. But we know that many histories are partial histories. Histories of war commonly leave out the role of women; histories of health and medicine commonly leave out the role of lay people in health and healing; histories of conflict commonly leave out the storyline of one's adversary.

And so local histories often emphasize their own local heroes and events, developing storylines that navigate between the tensions of challenges and champions. When loss becomes a theme it is treated as a temporary setback, or if it is not that, then simply tragedy. The enduring nature of loss, its influence on decision-making of many people, including the elite as well as the poor of any community, and the constructive building power of loss is seldom the framework or even major section in a social history.

Local governments, local historians or local community members could add to their local knowledge about themselves and their histories by re-examining, perhaps even rewriting their own histories to reflect and analyse the role of loss in their own life and times, and those of their ancestors. Such analyses provide a strong social understanding that death and loss are not only tragic and sad experiences but also sources of motivation, hope and creativity in people. Such a reminder is supportive of a constructive and normalizing understanding of death and loss, and helps restore balance not only to local histories but also self-understanding of life experience.

Building/architecture prize for carers

Many businesses and families are full-time carers. They conduct these activities in physical spaces that constrain and channel these social activities in set ways. The way bathrooms, entrances and kitchens are built frequently assumes able-body use. The way houses are designed frequently assumes use by nuclear families (two parents and two or three children). Extra rooms, such as playrooms (rumpus rooms), are designed for children to play under the watchful eye of parents. Parent 'retreats' are built so that older couples can have a recreational space away from teenagers, and their friends and video games, across the hall or downstairs.

Seldom are affordable homes designed so that certain rooms can convert easily into 'granny flats'; or bathrooms and kitchens designed for disabled as well as able-bodied use. The problem of stairs, outside gardens (instead of internal ones), walls that open out to the outside for access or viewing and recreation, and hidden but accessible internal support systems are just some of the possibilities and challenges for modern building design. The problem of serious illness and care is not an unusual circumstance. Disability is more usual than unusual. Most people will experience ageing. Housing designs that fail to accommodate these social realities are merely temporary housing for temporary experiences of life.

Equally, hospitals, hospices and nursing homes require serious rethinking. Part of the deserved stigma and negative press that institutions enjoy comes from the fact that many look like dormitories and prisons. Even those that attempt a 'home-like' look merely become 'home-like' dormitories and prisons. Surely there are architectural compromises or alternatives to the family home and the institution that are affordable to businesses and government. An annual building and architecture prize may well encourage those members of the community for whom building and designing is a life passion to rethink the problem of living design in the face of ageing and serious illness for public, private and domestic use.

Educational incentives for research into community support structures

A basic trophy or medallion costs no more than US$50–100. This is not big money, and yet prizes are prestigious, sought after and are valuable to career and identity. Local government and/or the local grief or palliative care agency can offer incentives to universities and colleges to encourage their students to examine possible community support structures for death, dying and loss.

Prizes offered to undergraduates for Best Student Essay or for Best Thesis by a graduate can be incentives for students to contribute to a community ideas about how to help itself in dying, death and loss. An educational institution is part of the community's social and intellectual capital and ALL faculties in those institutions have the time and resources to devote to some of these questions – in nursing, social sciences, social work, pastoral care, engineering, medicine, science and computing. Often a prize simply encourages people to think outside their own discipline's usual teaching concerns. A prize can be an important reminder to these educational institutions about the changing nature of their own community's priorities.

Encouraging research into community response, needs and support structures around matters to do with dying, death and loss, is also a way of assisting these institutions to set compassionate priorities themselves. It also helps encourage sustainability in compassionate initiatives by making compassionate priorities an ongoing concern of institutions beyond the local community, human services and local government.

Local 'sister city' exchanges

Sometimes, local communities may not have a significant number of people to create an exchange of information or support for each other. There may, for example, only be three or four families affected by motor neuron disease or dementia. These groups might be encouraged to set up 'Sister City' arrangements with a town of similar size. This works particularly well for small rural communities. A community of similar size and demographic characteristics can be chosen and contact made with people with similar experiences to hold an exchange day.

The people of one town who work with a family member with motor neuron disease may travel to that town for a weekend to exchange information about how they cope and conduct their care. In fact, the carers can meet at the same time, same venue, but different room, as the people living with motor neuron disease for whom they are caring. Both groups can benefit by meeting new people in their own situation.

Sometimes problem-solving can be more effective and new ideas about old situations might be developed. Networks and contacts can be pooled and new friends outside their own tight-knit community can be made. These 'Sister City' groups might also be 'virtual'. These groups can assemble over an Internet chat page at times convenient to both. Even in large cities, it can be useful to create interstate or intermunicipal networks for support. There may be few people one can or would want to link up with in the local area: people from another city may be more similar to your own social and cultural background than people from your own city or municipality.

Coalition for the universality of loss

A committee or subcommittee of three or four people can be established as part of any Compassionate City programme to monitor the print, radio and television media to promote better understanding about dying, death and loss, and to counter sectional understandings about loss. Examples might be that loss is greater for men at war than women who experience rape during that war, or that the grief experienced by dispossessed people is somehow less intense or traumatic than bereavement. It is important to note here that countering bias is NOT about arguing that all grief is the SAME but rather to take opportunities to broaden and contextualize the human experience of grief, so that listeners, viewers and readers can understand the universal NATURE of the experience rather then simply its circumstantial character.

Finally, monitoring the media should ensure a balance between fair coverage of the verities of dying, death and loss, and the ethical importance to families and communities of privacy, confidentiality and intrusion.

Weekly monitoring of newsprint stories can be commented on through submission of stories or letters-to-the-editor written by coalition members. Offers to speak on radio or TV programmes purporting to deal with certain illness experiences or loss can be accepted. Even more importantly, local newspapers might be encouraged to have a guest editorial about compassionate issues or to entertain a QA (question and answer) column that addresses anonymous readers' questions about dying, death and loss.

World spirituality show day

Once a year it will be useful to ask the community's religious adherents to ask their senior clerics to participate in promoting themselves to their local community. Few people will not benefit from knowing more about how religion acts as a living experience in the lives of so many of their community number. Even for humanists, atheists and hostile critics, such an annual event may help assuage prejudice, inform others of the nature and direction of the diverse spiritual traditions within the community, and introduce others to new ideas and services. None of this should imply or make for proselytizing of beliefs. In fact, preaching and 'selling' the beliefs of one's religion should be strictly avoided for the sake of community harmony and respect.

But such world spirituality show days should go beyond conventional religions such as Christianity and Buddhism for examples. Pagans, Spiritualists, Humanists, New Age religions and indigenous beliefs should be encouraged to showcase their ideas and practices. The main purpose of such 'showcasing' is to combat ignorance and hence ignorant responses from others. It will also be important to show how similar spiritual questions are provided for in diverse ways by different belief systems. Some religious systems are simply systems of worship while others contain health and medical models, occult practices or complex lifestyle prescriptions.

Only by understanding these systems do we offer ourselves greater choices in the storylines about the meaning of life and death and expand the horizons and opportunities for tolerance. Exactly how a world spirituality show day would look might vary enormously depending on how the main players wish it to look. However, a gathering at the local town hall with different rooms of displays and staffed tables of people who are willing to discuss the displays is a common practice. Although some churches will eschew the 'consumer-market' appearance of this style of public offering, other models are possible. The open gardens day system might be more dignified. Churches and gathering places of the different belief systems welcome everyone for an open day at their respective places all on the same day with different times and locations advertised in the local media. Whatever-ever model of show day is chosen such compassionate activities will promote greater curiousity, if not understanding, about diverse beliefs about the mysterious relationship between life and death.

Conclusion

Some of the above suggestions may be seen by readers as impractical, unwieldy or even laughable. The content of these suggestions is not designed to entertain the reader, or indeed to attract the reader's moral or professional approval. Professional and national sensibilities vary widely. As mentioned in the introduction to this chapter, all of these suggestions are meant to stimulate *your own ideas* – to modify the ones here or to replace them. Vardanega and Johnson (2002) have attempted to combine a Healthy Cities approach to grief and loss by producing user-friendly pamphlets to be used by a wide variety of community agencies. They emphasize, as I do here, that the facts of death and loss are a 'community's shared responsibility'. What works, or appears worthwhile, is worth trying.

These suggestions and many other public health events and activities should be read against the political and social wording of the four core Compassionate Cities ideas and the nine Compassionate Cities policy visions as these appear in Chapter 4. None of these action strategies has any real meaning outside of that policy context.

Furthermore, one should test each of your own or the community's ideas for social activities with a set of searching public health questions beginning with the following: what is the difference between a simple fun or novel social idea for community activity and a genuine public health activity?

To answer that question you should see if you can answer a few other related questions. In what way is the proposed activity a form of prevention, harm-minimization or early intervention for the troubles that death and loss can potentially bring to a community? In what ways do these activities genuinely arise out of partnerships within the community? In what ways are these activities sustainable, i.e. will outlive your personal or professional involvement with that community? In what ways do these activities target or alter the physical or social settings within the community for the better, i.e. for the betterment of support and information of everyone who encounters death and loss? In other words, how positively life-enhancing are these activities? Finally, how do you know these activities are doing what you hope for them?

Run your proposed activities past the big seven questions of public health and see if they really stack up as genuine health-promotion initiatives for end-of-life care in your community.

Box 11 Big seven checklist: Are the compassionate activities we promote public health ones?
You MUST be able to demonstrate ability in 1 OR 2 OR 3 PLUS 4–7

1   In what way do they help *PREVENT* social difficulties around dying, death, loss or care?
2   In what ways do they *HARM-MINIMIZE* difficulties we may not be able to prevent around dying, death, loss or care?
3   In what ways can these activities be understood as *EARLY INTERVENTIONS* along the journey of dying, death, loss or care?
4   In what way do these activities alter/change a *SETTING OR ENVIRONMENT* for the better in terms of our present or future responses to dying, death, loss or care?
5   In what ways are the proposed activities *PARTICIPATORY* – borne, partnered and nurtured by *community members*?
6   How *SUSTAINABLE* will these activities or programmes be without your future input?
7   How will we *EVALUATE* their success or usefulness so that we can justify their presence, their funding or their ongoing support?

Finally, three important points should be remembered when aspiring to success with these activities and events. Firstly, every attempt should be made to encourage *community ownership* of the events and activities. Police, schools, trade unions or clubs should be the lead agencies for these community actions. These are NOT suggestions for local government or professional services, though they may both be instrumental in suggesting, stimulating and supporting these activities.

Secondly, every activity should be designed, and its organizational personnel recruited, with an eye to the *sustainability* of the event or activity. One-off events do not carry learning or social value beyond one year and one audience. Think future. Think continuity of energy, interest and organizing responsibility.

And don't be sentimental about particular action strategies. Simple, modest but closely supported activities are more important to health promotion of a community than ideas that may appear more glamorous, high profile or require greater organizational skills. Start small. Aim for growth. Create compassion with small but sure steps.

Chapter 9

The future: a third-wave public health?

The first wave of public health policies and initiatives was associated with the promotion of clean drinking water, safer sewerage systems and building codes, and the control and isolation of infectious diseases. The emphasis in our first models of public health was firmly on disease prevention and containment. The second wave of policies and initiatives has frequently been developed in broader health-promotion terms. This has promoted health through education, legislation and communication around the morbidity and mortality of the modern lifestyle – obesity, chronic illnesses, work and road safety, tobacco and alcohol use, and so on. These second-wave initiatives, of which Healthy Cities are a key example, have been the subject of much recent criticism and reflection.

And there has been no shortage of this criticism. The future of public health has been the subject of significant and searching self-reflection and academic appraisal. How do compassionate ideas within a public health framework sit within that body of criticism? Do compassionate ideas simply complicate the 'new' public health by adding yet another social dimension to our ideas about community participation and social development? Can compassionate ideas address our concerns about the future of public health in the twenty-first century in the very terms that current public health writers themselves speak of them? In this final chapter I summarize the key reservations and challenges to the 'new' public health, and I argue that compassionate ideas, far from adding to our recent concerns and reservations, actually provide a useful and promising way forward. The ideas behind Compassionate Cities are an excellent redress of long-standing problems with the current and planned future directions of public health today.

Future challenges for public health

In a critical sociological tradition, Petersen and Lupton (1996: 174–80) identify three main problems with the new public health. First, they argue that despite an egalitarian rhetoric the new public health continues to identify what they term 'the contaminating other' (p 174). This is the sociological jargon for the communication and ideological style that divides people into 'pure' and 'polluted', or 'us' and 'them'. Consistently, public health experts identify problems in intellectual and social ways that position other people (apart from their good selves) as the 'problem population', e.g. slums, working-class areas, the gay and lesbian populations or Africa.

Public health approaches remain challenged by ideas about identities that integrate the notion that people change their identities as they move into different relationships and experience. The self as a changing, resisting, reflecting, future-oriented and intuitive agency challenges many of the new public health's most cherished assumptions of people as rational beings who desire health. Many people don't care for their own health; or don't articulate their priorities in these terms; or have health as one of a collection of priorities that are not particularly high, and is readily overtaken by other priorities and values.

Secondly, second-wave public health ideas shift the 'blame' for health problems from the individual to the community. While in the 1960s and 1970s an individual's habits of smoking or overeating were identified as contributing to their own subsequent illnesses, the new public health stressed the idea of partnerships. Partnerships between the individual, their community and the health services were ways that health could be promoted and maintained. Logically then, it could also be argued that 'failure' to be healthy now became a failure of these community partnerships. 'Communities' with higher morbidity and mortality rates may have lower rates of social capital, less access to services, less intersectoral collaboration, etc. These communities may 'not be working' in health terms. These scenarios and equations leave out the role of the government. This allows the language of the new public health to be used by cash-strapped or conservative governments to place the blame for poor health and participation rates on communities themselves rather than their own policies and funding priorities.

Thirdly, the new public health consistently fails to understand and respect the idea of resistance. Significant numbers of people resist public health imperatives and admonitions. Such resistance is often viewed as an extension of the problem of medical compliance and is seen as recalcitrance. Some people do love their cigarettes and their battered fish and chips. That's life. But the communication strategies frequently employed by national health-promotion campaigns can be a moral campaign directed at assaulting the character and not just the lifestyle of those who resist. This moralism has been aptly termed 'healthism' by Crawford (1980). Such healthism trivializes the language of respect for social and cultural differences and justifiably leads to charges about the 'gentrification of health'.

In a more health and medical practices tradition, Beaglehole and Bonita (1997: 229–32) argue that market economies have led to greater problems in international health and safety. This can be illustrated by the ease of passage and spread of mad cow disease, to problems of international violence, civil war and the mass migration of refugees. Furthermore, the growing ideology of individualism provides serious barriers to the desire for collective action required by so many public health policies.

The rise of AIDS and the reluctance by multinational pharmaceutical industries in wealthy countries to provide affordable treatments to the countries of Africa underline the important links between public health and human rights. Public health is no longer about immunization programmes at home but global equity and access. As Tulchinsky and Varavikova (2000) argue, the twenty-first century challenge for public health is its global mission. Whether for treatments, the rise of new infections or the control of old ones, what goes around, comes around.

Beaglehole and Bonita (1997) also observe that the rise and continuation of ethnic and religious rivalry fuels civil war and unrest, especially in Africa, the Middle East, and Central and Eastern Europe. There is a common inability of wealthy nations to link, let alone implicate, their own foreign policies to international attacks on them. There is also a tragic and ignorant habit of obfuscating the different violent responses to oppression, lack of international representation, racism, and chronic poverty and debt by employing the one-size-fits-all label of 'terrorism'. The failure of a searching and self-analysing social justice vision by wealthy nations is a serious barrier to global public health, both in the countries that breed militants for export and also to those wealthy countries whose citizens become the eventual targets of that violence.

A final challenge identified by Beaglehole and Bonita (1997) is the importance of moving towards broader rather than a more narrow, individualist focus for the future. We must look for broader political and cultural concepts that permit public health workers to rise above the narrow psychological ideas about individual behaviour and the equally narrow nationalism and self-interest of governments.

Tulchinsky and Varavikova (2000) argue that there is a pressing need to view the new public health in global terms. Global approaches to public health are essential if we are to contain the new infections, stem revival of some of the older ones, and tackle fundamental problems of economy and society that lie at the very heart of poor health for many countries. Furthermore, an important challenge for the second wave of public health initiatives is NOT to forget that most of the world – in fact about 77% – is still seriously involved in first-wave initiatives: combating infant and maternal deaths, malnutrition, poor population to resources ratios, infectious diseases, and environmental and disaster management.

Perhaps the ultimate challenge to the future of public health is a telling table that appears in Tulchinsky and Varavikova's (2000: 795) work that does not mention death or loss. This is the table listing all the World Health Organization (WHO) programmes currently on offer. Dying, death and loss – the universal human experiences – are absent from this list. WHO seems not to recognize the preventable social, physical, emotional or spiritual morbidity of living with disease that has no cure or of living with loss. The WHO is also not interested in the morbidity of loss for people who live with grief over their multiple experiences of endings in the context of death, dispossession or identity.

The final challenge for the future of public health is the establishment of even a basic recognition that death and loss are central public health matters.

Box 12 Challenges for the future of public health

- Overcome oppositional categories of health, lifestyle and identity
- Develop holistic political views of partnership inclusive of individuals, communities and governments
- Embrace concepts and practices about differences that are inclusive of dissent
- Recognize how market economies lead to additional dangers and risks to health, death and loss
- Overcome the ideology of individualism
- Understand that some matters to do with health, death and loss cannot be separated from human rights
- Embrace concepts that guide our practice broadly
- Recognize our interdependence internationally, domestically and emotionally
- The 'new' public health must not forget its commitment to the 'old' public health
- Recognize death and loss as fundamental human health issues

---

Third-wave public health: compassion and end-of-life care?

The ideas of 'compassion', 'the universality of death and loss' and the integration and recognition of 'death as an experience greater than physical demise', but inclusive of other important endings to identity and experience, provides the new public health with a clear, inclusive and practical way forward. Compassionate ideas and practices are the policy and practice basis for addressing the current limitations and challenges of the new public health, and may constitute a promising basis for a 'third wave' of public health initiatives in the twenty-first century. This might be a public health emphasis on inclusiveness based on *universal* human experiences of suffering and well-being and not simply categories of 'illness', 'disease' or 'health' states.

The idea of compassion is able to transcend and render irrelevant the old twentieth century categories of 'health' and 'welfare'. The public health expression of compassion may make these categories seamless and conterminous. Problems of economy and society, health and welfare, or law and moral conduct will be rearranged into a single discourse about the health, support and well-being of everyone. This will not simply be because some have fragile health, but because life itself is a fragile experience.

The ever-present experience of death and loss reminds us of our cultural, spiritual and political responsibilities towards one another because of their presence. And those reminders are not simply the mortality figures, as these emerge from any demography of death or epidemiology of disease, but rather, more pointedly and poignantly, in the *shared experiences* of death and loss themselves.

Only in seeing ourselves in the other through our own losses and finitude do we seriously attempt to erode the dispassionate public health gaze that reifies and abstractifies the 'other'. Only by seeing ourselves in the other do we seriously take up the challenge of emerging from a narcissistic and inward-looking individualism. Only when we understand our death and loss as the same as other people's experience of death and loss can we raise our eyes above the epidemiology to embrace the politics of health care. Only then, during these experiences of insight and empathy, do we truly understand our interdependence on each other in a deep social and emotional way that is lasting and strong.

If public health were truly searching for a broader framework of ideas to transcend the limited storylines of crisis counselling, health advertising, law enforcement and community surveillance, compassion opens up a set of conceptual and practice debates that meets the challenge of global health, social difference and solidarity. A commitment to compassion only reinforces a commitment to first-wave public health because we know that the toll of death and loss is greatest in countries where first-wave initiatives are needed. But more than this, we can learn from these countries what has almost been forgotten in many of the wealthier ones – that death *will* come no matter how many public health initiatives are developed. This is because all public health initiatives are ultimately about length and quality of life and not some mythical postponement of death itself.

Some countries might rediscover and trade the lessons learnt from their early or current health experiences. These lessons might be exchanged with other countries for the lessons those other countries might share from the community wisdom and empathy they have gained from experiencing much death and even great losses. These are public health lessons that bring a new international meaning to egalitarian ideas about equity, access, social development and aid for *all* nations, irrespective of their level of wealth.

Through the exchange of these ideas between the different corners of the global community, public health might recognize death and loss is not the only the reason why health is a central concern to all people. Mortal experiences themselves have crucial health implications for any social aspirations and planning for well-being. Important negative parts of the total human experience of death and loss are amenable to prevention and harm-minimization. Some of the positive lessons from the experiences of death and loss are amenable to support, enhancement and dissemination. This work cannot begin unless we take up the challenge of integrating these human experiences into our intellectual and political agendas and our international and local health organizations. We need to start this process now.

The end?

Can there be any doubt that we live in strange times? Often it seems to me as if one half of the modern world believes it will never die. Death is increasingly being greeted in wealthy countries and communities with more than mere shock or horror. Death is no longer a taboo subject but it is now commonly viewed as a great social rudeness. The violence and finality of death is an affront to everything we value – planning, certainty, cerebral abstractions and reliable help. For the other half of the world, the poorest parts of the world, death is so common, so ever present, that its appearance seems to be less important than other less common experiences in life – safety, dignity, autonomy, food, national sovereignty and freedom from dangerous enemies. These things seem more and more important than death itself to more and more people who experience the infrequent and precarious quality of these other issues.

And even in Australia, Europe or the USA there is frequently an inexplicable and irreconcilable difference in the experience of those who worry about their next career move or golf day and those for whom life is just an empty word since the death of their only child. Those who know this kind of experience of bereavement, who know the emptiness of the heart that comes with deep loss, also partly understand the loss of country and identity that comes from the refugee, colonial or dementia experience, even if they are not literate about the relevant histories or biographies of those concerned. After all, loss is loss.

These widespread experiences of endings, and the losses that inevitably emerge in their wake, are the most important potential basis of our interpersonal and international connection with one another. We can only kill if we cannot feel the killing. The compassion we offer one another can only be equitable and unwavering if this arises from a genuine empathy. The integration of death and loss into our global public health concerns is the one important linkage that we must eventually make if we are to draw on the experiences that unite us. To make those steps possible we must restore the idea and practice of compassion to its rightful place – at the very top of our public health priorities.

References

Abel, E.K. (1986) The hospice movement: Institutionalizing innovation, *International Journal of Health Services* 16(1): 71–85.

Adamolekun, K. (1999) Bereavement salutations among the Yorubas of Western Nigeria, *Omega* 39(4): 277–85.

Aicher, J. (1998) *Designing Healthy Cities: Prescriptions, principles and practice.* Malabar, Florida: Krieger.

Anthias, F. and Yuval-Davis, N. (1992) *Racialized Boundaries.* London: Routledge.

Aries, P. (1974) *Western Attitudes Toward Death.* London: Marion Boyars.

Armstrong, D. (1987) Silence and truth in death and dying, *Social Science & Medicine* 24(8): 651–7.

Ashton, J., Grey, P. and Barnard, K. (1986) Healthy Cities – WHO's new public health initiative, *Health Promotion* 1(3): 319–24.

Bank-Mikkelsen, N. (1980) 'Denmark', in R.J. Flynn & K.E. Nitsch (eds), *Normalisation, Social Integration and Community Services*, Austin, Texas.

Barnhart, R.K. (ed.) (1988) *The Barnhart Dictionary of Etymology.* New York: H.W. Wilson and Co.

Baum, F. (1993) Healthy Cities and change: Social movement or bureaucratic tool?, *Health Promotion International* 8(1): 31–40.

Baum, F. (1998) *The New Public Health: An Australian perspective.* Melbourne: Oxford University Press.

Baum, F. (1999) Social capital: Is it good for your health?, *Journal of Epidemiology and Community Health* 53(4): 195–6.

Bauman, Z. (1992) *Mortality, Immortality and Other Life Strategies.* Cambridge: Polity Press.

Beaglehole, R. and Bonita, R. (1997) *Public Health at the Crossroads: Achievements and prospects.* Cambridge: Cambridge University Press.

Beck, U. (1992) *Risk Society: Towards a new modernity.* London: Sage.

Becker, E. (1973) *The Denial of Death.* New York: Macmillan.

Beilharz, P. (2000) *Zygmunt Bauman: Dialectic of modernity.* London: Sage.

Bourdieu, P. (1980) Le capital social: Notes provisoires, *Actes de la recherche en Sciences Sociales*, 31: 2–3.

Bourne, J. (1987) *Homelands of the mind: Jewish feminism and identity politics*, Race and class pamphlet No. 1. London: Institute of Race Relations.

Bradshaw, A. (1996) The spiritual dimension of hospice: The secularization of an ideal, *Social Science and Medicine* 43(3): 409–19.

Breslow, L. (2002) *The Encyclopedia of Public Health* (four volumes). New York: Macmillan Reference USA.

Brown, H. and Smith, H. (1992) 'Assertion, not assimilation: A feminist perspective on the normalisation principle', in H. Brown and H. Smith (eds) *Normalisation: A reader for the nineties*. London: Routledge.

Buckingham, R.W. (1983) *The Complete Hospice Guide*. New York: Harper Colophon Books.

Carey, J. (ed.) (1999) *The Faber Book of Utopias*. London: Faber and Faber.

Carroll, J. and Manne, R. (eds) (1992) *Shutdown: The failure of economic rationalism and how to rescue Australia*. Melbourne: Text Publishing.

Cassell, C.K. and Demel, B. (2001) Remembering death: public policy in the USA, *Journal of the Royal Society of Medicine* 94(9): 433–6.

Castells, M. (1996) *The Rise of the Network Society*. Oxford: Blackwell.

Castells, M. (1997) *The Power of Identity*. Oxford: Blackwell.

Castells, M. (1998) *End of the Millenium*. Oxford: Blackwell.

Catford, J. (1999) WHO is making a difference through health promotion, *Health Promotion International* 14(1): 1–4.

Clark, D. (1999) Cradled to the grave? Terminal care in the United Kingdom, 1948–67, *Mortality* 4(3): 225–47.

Clark, D. (2000) Palliative care history: A ritual process?, *European Journal of Palliative Care* 7(2): 50–5.

Coleman, J. (1988) Social capital in the creation of human capital, *American Journal of Sociology* 94 (Suppl): S95–S120.

Council of Europe (1995) *Tackling Racism and Xenophobia: Practical action at the local level*. Strasbourg: Council of Europe Press.

Cox, F.M., Erlich, J.L., Rothman, J. and Tropman, J.E. (1984) *Tactics and Techniques of Community Practice*. Itasca, Illinois: Peacock Publishers.

Crawford, R. (1980) Healthism and the medicalisation of everyday life, *International Journal of Health Services* 10(3): 365–89.

Crisp, B., Swerissen, H. and Duckett, S. (2000) Four approaches to capacity building in health: consequences for measurement and accountability, *Health Promotion International* 15(2): 99–107.

Crow, G. and Allan, G. (1994) *Community life: An introduction to local social relations*. Hertfordshire: Harvester-Wheatsheaf.

Dalley, G. (1992) 'Social welfare ideologies and normalisation: links and conflicts', in H. Brown and H. Smith (eds) *Normalisation: A reader for the nineties*. London: Routledge.

Detels, R., Holland, W.H., McEwen, J. and Omen, G.S. (1997) *The Oxford Textbook of Public Health* (three volumes). New York: Oxford University Press.

Dooris, M. (1999) Healthy Cities and local agenda 21: the UK experiences – challenges for the new millennium, *Health Promotion International* 14(4): 365–75.

Dubos, R. (1959) *Mirage of Health*. New York: Doubleday.

Dudgeon, D.J., Robertas, R.F., Doerner, K. et al. (1995) When does palliative care begin? A needs assessment of cancer patients with recurrent disease, *Journal of Palliative Care* 11: 5–9.

Duhl, R (1986) The Healthy City: Its function and future, *Health Promotion* 1(1): 55–60.

Eaton, R. (2000) 'The city as an intellectual exercise', in R. Schaer, G. Claeys and L.T. Sargent (eds) *Utopia: The search for the ideal society in the Western world.* New York: Oxford University Press, pp 119–31.

Elias, N. (1985) *The Loneliness of Dying.* Oxford: Blackwell.

Emerson, E. (1992) 'What is normalisation?', in H. Brown and H. Smith (eds) *Normalisation: A reader for the nineties.* London: Routledge.

Fine, B. (2001) *Social Capital versus Social Theory.* London: Routledge.

Finlay, I.G. and Jones, R.V.H. (1995) Definitions in palliative care [letter], *British Medical Journal* 311: 754.

Fook, J. (2002) *Social Work: critical theory and practice.* London: Sage.

Fraser, M. (1997) 'The legacy of suicide: The impact of suicide on families', in K. Charmaz, G. Howarth and A. Kellehear (eds) *The Unknown Country: Death in Australia, Britain and the USA.* New York: St Martin's Press, pp 58–71.

Friedson, E. (1971) *Professional Dominance: The social structure of medical care.* Chicago: Aldine.

Fryback, P.B. (1993) Health for people with a terminal diagnosis, *Nursing Science Quarterly* 6(3): 147–59.

Fryer, P. (1988) A Healthy City strategy 3 years on – the case of Oxford City Council, *Health Promotion* 3(2): 213–17.

Funk, I.K. (ed.) (1963) *Funk and Wagnalls New Standard Dictionary of the English Language.* New York: Funk and Wagnalls.

Giddens, A. (1991) *Modernity and Self-identity: Self and society in the late modern age.* Cambridge: Polity Press.

Giddens, A. (1998) *The Third Way: The renewal of social democracy.* Cambridge: Polity Press.

Giddens, A. (2000) *The Third Way and its Critics.* Cambridge: Polity Press.

Gillis, J.R. (ed.) (1994) *Commemorations: The politics of national identity.* Princeton, NJ: Princeton University Press.

Gottfried, R.S. (1983) *The Black Death.* New York: Macmillan.

Gray, R.E. (2001) Cancer self-help groups are here to stay: Issues and challenges for health professionals, *Journal of Palliative Care* 17(1): 53–8.

Groopman, J. (2004) Annals of Medicine. The Grief Industry: How much does crisis counselling help – or hurt?, *The New Yorker*, January 26: pp 30–8.

Hancock, T. (1993) 'The Healthy City from concept to application', in J.K. Davies and M.P. Kelly (eds) *Healthy Cities: Research and practice.* London: Routledge.

Hancock, T. and Dahl, L. (1985) *Healthy Cities: promoting health in the urban context.* WHO, Copenhagen: Healthy Cities Symposium, Lisbon.

Henley, N. and Donovan, R.J. (1999) Threat appeals in social marketing: Death as a 'special case', *International Journal of Nonprofit and Voluntary Sector Marketing* 4(4): 300–19.

Herlihy, D. (1997) *The Black Death and the Transformation of the West.* Cambridge: Harvard University Press.

Homan, M.S. (1999) *Promoting Community Change: making it happen in the real world.* Pacific Grove, California: Brooks/Cole Publishing Co.

Ife, J. (1995) *Community Development: Creating community alternatives – vision, analysis and practice.* South Melbourne: Longman.

Illich, I. (1976) *Limits to Medicine.* Harmondsworth: Penguin.

Institute of Medicine (1997) *Approaching Death: Improving care at the end of life.* Washington, DC: National Academy Press.

Jenks, C. (ed.) (1993) *Cultural Reproduction.* London: Routledge.

Jewson, N.D. (1976) The disappearance of the sick man from medical cosmology, 1770–1870, *Sociology* 10: 225–44.

Kearl, M. (1989) *Endings: A sociology of death and dying.* New York: Oxford University Press.

Kellehear, A. (1984) Are we a 'death denying' society? A sociological review, *Social Science and Medicine* 18(9): 713–23.

Kellehear, A. (1996) *Experiences Near Death: Beyond medicine and religion.* New York: Oxford University Press.

Kellehear, A. (1998) Guest editorial: Death, sociology and public health in Australia, *Mortality* 3(2): 109–10.

Kellehear, A. (1999a) *Health Promoting Palliative Care.* Melbourne: Oxford University Press.

Kellehear, A. (1999b) Health promoting palliative care: Developing a social model for practice, *Mortality* 4(1): 75–82.

Kellehear, A. (2000a) 'The Australian way of death: Formative historical and social influences', in A. Kellehear (ed.) *Death and Dying in Australia.* Melbourne: Oxford University Press, pp 1–13.

Kellehear, A. (2000b) Spirituality and palliative care: a model of needs, *Palliative Medicine* 14(2): 144–55.

Kellehear, A. (2002) Grief and loss: Past, present and future, *Medical Journal of Australia* 177: 176–7.

Kellehear, A. (2003) 'Public health challenges in the care of the dying', in P. Liamputtong and H. Gardner (eds) *Health, Social Change and Communities.* Melbourne: Oxford University Press, 88–99.

Kellehear, A. (2004) Public health approaches to palliative care: Developments in Australia, *Rikkyo Social Work Review* 23: 27–35.

Kellehear, A., Rumbold, B. and Bateman, G. (2003) *Practice guidelines for health promoting palliative care.* Melbourne: Palliative Care Unit, La Trobe University.

Kendall, A. (1970) *Medieval Pilgrims,* London: Wayland.

Kenny, S. (1999) *Developing Communities for the Future: Community development in Australia.* Melbourne: Nelson.

Kuhn, T. (1962) *The Structure of Scientific Revolutions.* Chicago: University of Chicago Press.

Lin, N., Cook, K. and Burt, R.S. (2001) *Social Capital: Theory and research.* New York: Aldine de Gruyter.

Lynn, J. (2002) 'Improving care of the "dying"', in V. Yeoman, M. Box and C. Papadopoulos (eds) *Challenges to improving the care of the dying,* conference papers of the third Victorian Conference in Palliative Care. Melbourne: Palliative Care Victoria, pp 1–20.

Maclean, M. and Grove, D. (eds) (1991) *Women's Issues in Social Policy.* London: Routledge.

Mayo, M. (1994) *Communities and Caring: The mixed economy of welfare.* London: Macmillan.

Mayo, M. (2000) *Cultures, Communities, Identities: Cultural strategies for participation and empowerment.* Basingstoke: Palgrave.

McGill, P. and Emerson, E. (1992) 'Normalisation and applied behaviour analysis: values and technology in human services', in H. Brown and H. Smith (eds) *Normalisation: A reader for the nineties*. London: Routledge.

McKeown, T. (1971) 'A historical appraisal of the medical task', in G. McLachlan and T. McKeown (eds) *Medical History and Medical Care*. London: Oxford University Press.

McManners, J. (1985) *Death and the Enlightenment*. Oxford: Oxford University Press.

Najman, J. (2000) 'The demography of death: Patterns of Australian mortality', in A. Kellehear (ed.) *Death and Dying in Australia*. Melbourne: Oxford University Press.

New Society (1988) *Grassroots Initiatives: A selection from New Society*. London: Bedford Square Press.

Nirje, B. (1970) The normalisation principle: implications and comments, *Journal of Mental Subnormality* 16: 62–70.

North, M. (1972) *The Secular Priests: Psychotherapists in contemporary society*. Sydney: George, Allen and Unwin.

Onions, C.T. (ed.) (1966) *The Oxford Dictionary of English Etymology*. London: Oxford University Press.

Ottawa Charter for Health Promotion (1986) *Health Promotion*, 1: iii–v.

Palliative Care Australia (2003) *Palliative Care Service Provision in Australia: A planning guide*, 2nd end. Canberra: Palliative Care Australia. (ISBN 0 9578342 92 [www.pallcare.org.au])

Partridge, E. (1958) *Origins: A short etymological dictionary of modern English*. London: Routledge and Kegan Paul.

Petersen, A. and Lupton, D. (1996) *The New Public Health: Health and self in the age of risk*. Sydney: Allen and Unwin.

Platt, C. (1996) *King Death: The Black Death and its aftermath in late-medieval England*. Toronto: University of Toronto Press.

Porter, R.R. (1972) *The contribution of the biological and medical sciences to human welfare*. Presidential address of the British Association for the Advancement of Science. Swansea Meeting. Published 1971 by the British Association, p 95.

Powles, J. (1973) On the limitations of modern medicine, *Science, Medicine and Man* 1: 1–30.

Putnam, R.D. (1993) *Making Democracy Work: civic traditions in modern Italy*. Princeton, NJ: Princeton University Press.

Putter, A.M. (1997) *The Memorial Rituals Book for Healing and Hope*. Amityville, NY: Baywood Publishing Co.

Radest, H.B. (1990) *The Devil and Secular Humanism: The children of the enlightenment*. New York: Praeger Publishers.

Raphael, B. (1986) *When disaster strikes: How individuals and communities cope with catastrophe*. New York: Basic Books.

Rees, S. (1995) 'The fraud and the fiction', in S. Rees and G. Rodley (eds) *The Human Costs of Managerialism*. Sydney: Pluto Press, pp 15–27.

Rees, S. and Rodley, G. (eds) (1995) *The Human Costs of Managerialism*. Sydney: Pluto Press.

Rumbold, B. (1998) 'Implications of mainstreaming hospice into palliative care services', in J.M. Parker and S. Aranda (eds) *Palliative Care: Explorations and challenges*. Sydney: Maclennon and Petty, pp 3–20.

Schopenhauer, A. (1942) 'The art of literature', in *Complete Essays of Schopenhauer: Seven books in one volume* [translated, T. Bailey Saunders]. New York: Wiley Book Co.

Seale, C. (1998) *Constructing Death: The sociology of dying and bereavement.* Cambridge: Cambridge University Press.

Sennett, R. (1994) *Flesh and Stone: The body and the city in Western civilisation.* New York: W.W. Norton and Co.

Sheldon, F.M. (2000) Dimensions of the role of the social worker in palliative care, *Palliative Medicine* 14: 491–8.

St Leger, L. (1997) Health promoting settings: from Ottawa to Jakarta, *Health Promotion International* 12(2): 99–102.

Starr, P. (1982) *The Social Transformation of American Medicine.* New York: Basic Books.

Sumption, J. (1975) *Pilgrimage: An image of mediaeval religion.* Totowa, NJ: Rowman and Littlefield.

Szivos, S. (1992) 'The limits to integration', in H. Brown and H. Smith (eds) *Normalisation: A reader for the nineties.* London: Routledge.

Task Force on Palliative Care, Last Acts Campaign, Robert Woods Johnson Foundation (1998) Precepts in palliative care, *Journal of Palliative Care* 1(2): 109–12.

Thompson, J.W. (1928) *Economic and Social History of the Middle Ages (300–1300): Volume 1.* New York: Frederick Unger Publishing Co.

Thomson, M., Rose, C., Wainwright, W. et al. (2001) Activities of counsellors in a hospice/palliative care environment, *Journal of Palliative Care* 17(4): 229–35.

Torrens, P. (1978) *The American Health Care Delivery System: Issues and problems.* St Louis: C.V Mosby.

Tsouros, A.D. (1990) *World Health Organization Healthy Cities project: A project becomes a movement.* Copenhagen: WHO Project Office, FADL Publishers.

Tsouros, A.D. (1995) The WHO Healthy Cities project: state of the art and future plans, *Health Promotion International* 10(2): 133–41.

Tulchinsky, T.H. and Varavikova, E.A. (2000) *The New Public Health: An introduction for the 21st century.* London: Academic Press.

Turner, B.S. (ed.) (1993) *Citizenship and Social Theory.* London: Sage.

Turner, B.S. and Rojek, C. (2001) *Society and Culture: Principles of scarcity and solidarity.* London: Sage.

Vafiadis, P (2001) *Palliative Medicine.* Sydney: McGraw-Hill.

Vardanega, L. and Johnson, A. (2002) Coping with grief and loss: A community's shared responsibility, *Australian Journal of Primary Health* 8(3): 100–5.

Waddington, I. (1973) The role of the hospital in the development of modern medicine: A sociological analysis, *Sociology* 7(2): 211–24.

Walter, T. (1991) Modern death – taboo or not taboo?, *Sociology* 25(2): 293–310.

Walter, T. (1994) *The Revival of Death.* London: Routledge.

Wellman, B. and Wortley, S. (1990) Different strokes from different folks: Community ties and social support, *American Journal of Sociology* 96(3): 558–88.

Whaley, J. (ed) (1981) *Mirrors of Mortality.* London: Europa Publications Ltd.

Whitehead, S. (1992) 'The social origins of normalisation', in H. Brown and H. Smith (eds) *Normalisation: A reader for the nineties.* London: Routledge.

Williams, F. (1989) *Social Policy: A critical introduction*. Cambridge: Polity Press.

Willis, E. (1989) *Medical Dominance*. Sydney: Allen & Unwin.

Wolfensberger, W. (1975) *The Origin and Nature of our Institutional Models*. Syracuse, NY: Human Policy Press.

Wolfensberger, W. (1992) *A brief introduction to social role valorization*, revised edn. Syracuse, NY: Training Institute for Human Service Planning, Leadership and Change Agency (Syracuse University).

World Health Organization (1986) Ottawa charter for health promotion, *Health Promotion* 1(4): i–v.

World Health Organization (1996) *Creating Healthy Cities in the 21ˢᵗ Century*. Geneva: WHO.

Ziegler, P. (1969) *The Black Death*. Harmondsworth: Penguin.

Index